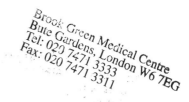

Research Opportunities
in Primary Care

Edited by

Yvonne Carter
and
Cathryn Thomas

Foreword by

John Swales
*Director of Research and
Development, NHS*

Radcliffe Medical Press

Radcliffe Medical Press Ltd
18 Marcham Road, Abingdon, Oxon OX14 1AA

British Library Cataloguing in Publication Data

A catalogue record for this book is available from the British Library.

ISBN 1 85775 242 2

Typeset by Advance Typesetting Ltd, Oxfordshire
Printed and bound by the Alden Press, Oxford.

Contents

Foreword

The ability to live with change has become a necessity for all those involved in the formidable enterprise we call the health service. Two types of challenge face us. The pace of discovery and innovation tests all of us, in some cases almost to destruction. But we also have to live with social changes in the way in which care is delivered within the health service and the high public expectations of what is offered.

Primary care is at the eye of the storm. The move towards a primary care-led NHS in some ways only acknowledges an inescapable fact. Most of the advice, support and treatment which an individual gets from the health service will begin and end with primary care. If what is on offer is inappropriate or of poor quality, the consequences will be far-reaching and often irrecoverable. Society has a right to expect that care is informed by robust and relevant evidence. Some of that evidence may be generalisable from other countries or from other fields of work. In other cases, the original research has to be carried out in primary care. This is obviously true of the way in which care is delivered. As Denis Pereira Gray has been telling us for some time, there is also a world of difference between the average patient seen in general practice and the rather atypical patient who volunteers to enter the artificial environment of a randomised controlled trial.

The accumulation and analysis of relevant scientific evidence is a difficult and painstaking job. It is also enormously exciting. The level of enthusiasm for research-based evidence in the face of so many other pressures and difficulties is one of the most encouraging features of the present scene. That is why the NHS research and development programme is committed to a strategic development in primary care involving a doubling of investment over the next five years. We are not making everyone into a researcher, although we have a pressing need to increase the numbers who are participating actively in research. We are attempting, and there is evidence that we are succeeding, to change the culture to one in which all professionals question the appropriateness of what they are doing. Asking the right question is just as important as finding the answer.

Yvonne Carter and Cathryn Thomas have assembled a formidable list of contributors in their innovative enterprise. The range of professional and scientific skills they exhibit underlines the collaborative nature of modern successful science.

Their powerful credentials are reasons for optimism in a field where numbers are still small, although growing. This book will, I am sure, help that process not only by instruction and guidance, but also by transmitting some of that transparent enthusiasm which characterises work which is both intellectually challenging and of great value.

Professor John Swales
October 1998

Preface

'Research has been called good business, a necessity, a gamble, a game. It is none of these – it's a state of mind.' Martin H Fischer: Fischerisms (Howard Fabing and Ray Marr).

Much has been written about improving the research capacity in primary care. Health professionals in primary care are being encouraged to play a more active role in research, with improved access to funding, but many are unsure how or where to start. The dilemma of whether research is only for enthusiasts or for all continues. This book is designed to introduce the reader to a range of research opportunities relevant to primary healthcare teams. The aim is to create a set of practical notes complemented by specific examples of community-based activity that are attractive to read and stimulate personal reflection. Each chapter outlines the history and philosophy behind the various developments then deals with the day-to-day aspects of research. The final section of many chapters is written by people who are actually doing research in this setting to give a 'hands-on' feel of what it means in practical terms. Discovering the pitfalls and the successes from 'grassroots' practitioners will, we hope, also help to bring reality to the work. It is anticipated that this new work will complement *Research Methods in Primary Care*, edited by the same team.

Academic general practice is now established in every undergraduate medical school in the United Kingdom. Many departments are providing teaching on research methods with an increasing number of diploma courses and masters degrees being developed for postgraduate students. New posts are being created for GP registrars and young principals with protected time for personal development and research. General practice-based research networks are gaining support and momentum around the UK. The future appointment and possible 'accreditation' of formally recognised research practices can only increase both the quality and quantity of research in general practice and primary care. The opportunities are numerous and we hope that this book will help readers know which one suits them and their situation best.

The editors are both practising GPs who also hold senior academic posts in two University Departments of General Practice. We have substantial teaching experience in relation to research methods teaching. The contributors have been selected for particular areas of interest and expertise. The book describes the research work undertaken recently by GPs and other professionals in a variety of primary care settings. It gives information on a range of options for individuals and practice teams who want to be involved in research: everything from being part of a primary care research network to undertaking a higher degree. At present there is no easy way for an 'ordinary' primary care professional who is interested in research to find out about what it is really like to be involved without contacting someone who is already doing it. This may be difficult as it involves a certain commitment even to declare an interest. The individual may not know who to ask. This book offers a unique opportunity to read what impact being part of the MRC General Practice Research Framework, or a research active practice, or doing a higher degree has on the professional and practice involved.

Our intended readership is wide and includes GPs and members of the primary healthcare team, particularly practice and community nurses, GP registrars and pharmacists. We hope that the editors' and authors' enthusiasm for research will be infectious to our readers, stimulating an enjoyment of research in primary care.

Yvonne Carter
Cathryn Thomas
October 1998

List of contributors

CHAPTER 1

Professor Denis Pereira Gray
Professor of General Practice
Institute of General Practice
Exeter Postgraduate Medical Centre

CHAPTER 2

Professor Pali Hungin
General Practitioner
Cleveland

Professor Tony Kendrick
Head of Department
Department of Primary Medical Care
University of Southampton

Dr Michael Moore
General Practitioner
Salisbury

Felicity Thompson
Practice Nurse
Salisbury

CHAPTER 3

Dr Madge Vickers
Coordinator of Medical Research
    Council General Practice
    Research Framework
The Wolfson Institute of Preventative
    Medicine
London

Lesley Hand
Practice Nurse Manager
The Beeches Health Centre
Bungay

Dr Christopher Hand
Associate Advisor
General Practice Unit
School of Health Policy and Practice
University of East Anglia

CHAPTER 4

Dr Jim Cox
General Practitioner
Cumbria

Dr Andrew Farmer
General Practitioner
Thame

Dr David Seamark
Lecturer
Institute of General Practice
Exeter Postgraduate Medical
　School

CHAPTER 5

Professor Bonnie Sibbald
Professor of Health Services
　Research
National Primary Care Research and
　Development Centre
University of Manchester

Dr Helen Lester
Clinical Research Fellow
Department of General Practice
The Medical School
University of Birmingham

Dr Jonathan Graffy
General Practitioner
London

CHAPTER 6

Dr Douglas Fleming
Director of Birmingham Research Unit
Royal College of General Practitioners
Birmingham

Dr Norman Smith
General Practitioner
Birmingham

Dr Andy Ross
General Practitioner
Birmingham

CHAPTER 7

Professor Philip Hannaford
Chair of Primary Care
RCGP Centre for Primary Care
　Research and Epidemiology
Department of General Practice and
　Primary Care
University of Aberdeen

CHAPTER 8

Dr Tony Avery
Senior Lecturer
Department of General Practice
University of Nottingham

Professor Yvonne Carter
Head of Department
Department of General Practice and
　Primary Care
Queen Mary & Westfield College
University of London

Dr Amanda Howe
Senior Lecturer
Department of General Practice
Northern General Hospital
Sheffield

CHAPTER 9

Dr Cathryn Thomas
Senior Lecturer
Department of General Practice
The Medical School
University of Birmingham

Dr Nicky Britten
Senior Lecturer
Department of General Practice &
　Primary Care
Guy's, Kings & St Thomas's Hospitals

Dr Graham Calvert
Lecturer
Department of General Practice &
    Primary Care
Guy's, Kings & St Thomas's Hospitals

Dr Roland Petchey
Lecturer
Department of General Practice
University of Nottingham

Norma O'Flynn
Principal in General Practice
Department of General Practice &
    Primary Care
Guy's, Kings & St Thomas's Hospitals

Dr Adrian Freeman
Research Fellow
Institute of General Practice
Postgraduate Medical School
Exeter

CHAPTER 10

Dr Ross Taylor
Senior Lecturer
Department of General Practice &
    Primary Care
University of Aberdeen

Fenny Green
Research Administrator
Royal College of General
    Practitioners

Professor Bonnie Sibbald
Professor of Health Services Research
National Primary Care Research and
    Development Centre
University of Manchester

Dr Chris Butler
Lecturer
Department of General Practice
University of Wales College of
    Medicine
Cardiff

Dr Charlotte Paterson
General Practitioner
Taunton

CHAPTER 11

Dr John Campbell
Senior Lecturer
Department of General Practice
Guy's, Kings & St Thomas's Hospitals

Alison Wilson
Nurse Coordinator
Fisher Medical Centre
Skipton

CHAPTER 12

Dr Brenda Leese
Senior Research Fellow
National Primary Care Research and
    Development Centre
University of Manchester

Dr Jackie Bailey
Research Associate
Department of Public Health &
    Epidemiology
University of Newcastle upon Tyne

Ann Mahon
Fellow in Health Services
Health Services Management Unit
Manchester

CHAPTER 13

Dr Alastair Wright
Editor of the *British Journal of General Practice*
Royal College of General Practitioners

Dr Joe Kai
Lecturer
Department of General Practice
University of Newcastle upon Tyne

CHAPTER 14

Dr Norman Beale
General Practitioner
Wiltshire

CHAPTER 15

Dr Martin Underwood
Senior Lecturer
Department of General Practice and Primary Care
Queen Mary & Westfield College

Professor Yvonne Carter
Head of Department
Department of General Practice and Primary Care
Queen Mary & Westfield College

Dr David Fitzmaurice
Senior Lecturer
Department of General Practice
University of Birmingham

Dr Johanna Cornwell
Academic Fellow
Department of General Practice and Primary Care
Queen Mary & Westfield College

CHAPTER 16

Dr Chris Griffiths
Senior Lecturer
Department of General Practice and Primary Care
Queen Mary & Westfield College

Dr Gene Feder
Senior Lecturer
Department of General Practice and Primary Care
Queen Mary & Westfield College

CHAPTER 17

Professor Fiona Ross
Professor of Primary Care Nursing
Faculty of Healthcare Science
St George's Hospital Medical School

Margaret Elliott
Professional Development Nurse
Camden & Islington Community NHS Trust

CHAPTER 18

Dr Geoffrey Harding
Senior Lecturer
Department of General Practice and Primary Care
Queen Mary & Westfield College

Dr Kevin Taylor
Senior Lecturer
School of Pharmacy
University of London

CHAPTER 19

Dr Madeleine Gantley
Senior Lecturer
Department of General Practice and Primary Care
Queen Mary & Westfield College

Dr Geoffrey Harding
Senior Lecturer
Department of General Practice and Primary Care
Queen Mary & Westfield College

1

Research in general practice

Denis Pereira Gray

HISTORY

The history of research in general practice and primary care goes back at least to the end of the 18th century. In those days, the medical profession was not as strictly divided as it is now and doctors could and did move between generalist and specialist medicine, essentially between being a general practitioner and being a physician or surgeon, and sometimes both at once.

Thoughtful general practitioners could and did not only see research opportunities but pursued them with such effect that several of them contributed knowledge of world-class importance. Jenner, at the end of the 18th century, studied smallpox in rural Gloucestershire. From his experiments with vaccination with cowpox he was able to show protection against the disease and in effect led an initiative which 200 years later has enabled smallpox to be eliminated worldwide.

In the 1840s William Budd, working in a rural practice in mid-Devon, researched the pattern of spread of typhoid and typhus and was the first person to separate the two. Budd later moved to Bristol but his book *Typhoid Fever* became a classic and led to him becoming an FRS.[1]

Sir James Mackenzie, in a working class practice in Burnley in Lancashire, became the world's leading authority on the rhythm of the heart,[2] which he researched using an instrument he invented called the polygraph. This was the forerunner of the ECG machine.

In the 20th century, William Pickles (1939), in a rural practice in Wensleydale, Yorkshire, researched the pattern of infectivity of some common diseases and what came to be called Bornholm disease.[3] After the Second World War, Crombie,[4] Fry[5] and Tudor Hart[6] were among the outstanding single-practice researchers. The era of the university departments then took over, with Stott and West,[7] Kinmonth, Angus and Baum[8] and Howie, Heaney and Maxwell[9] among the leading contributors.

RATIONALE FOR RESEARCH IN GENERAL PRACTICE

The reasons for doing research in general practice/primary care, and doing much more of it, are clear and strong. However, because general practice does not have a formal research training programme and because in the past most research in medicine has been undertaken in laboratories and hospitals, it is necessary to set out the reasons briefly.

Needs of the population

In the British, Dutch and some other systems of healthcare, patients first seek advice from their GPs and a proportion of them are then referred to specialists. In the UK, this proportion is 13%, which means that 87% of patients receive all their care in primary care.[10]

Unique field

The first important reason for a good deal of research being done in primary care is that there is a whole range of conditions, including most of the common infections and most of the common disturbances of mental state, which are not normally referred to hospital at all. It follows that if research is undertaken only with secondary care leadership these important problems from which patients suffer will not be adequately researched or even researched at all.

Second, laboratories and hospitals are essentially specialist institutions. They are organised by people who have developed great expertise, but in a narrow field. Specialist research of this kind has been responsible for most of the major contributions to medical knowledge and it needs to continue. However, the other side of the coin of specialism is loss of breadth and it is the particular contribution of the generalist to provide breadth and balance in medical practice. Appropriate research and research funding needs to go on whole-person medicine.[11]

The third reason is the nature of society and family life. It is extremely difficult to research medico-social issues unless one is personally familiar with them and has first-hand experience of them. Thus problems to do with the family, family relationships, doctor–patient relationships, continuity of care, and many aspects of social deprivation and the environment are all more logically researched in primary rather than in secondary or tertiary care.

THE DEVELOPMENT OF GENERAL PRACTICE

Despite the world-class contributions of GPs in the 18th and 19th centuries, the quantity and quality of research in the 20th century has been disappointing. In order to plan and maximise both quality and quantity it is necessary to understand the reasons for the state of general practice research[12] and to plan carefully to develop it in the future. Three obstacles have dogged general practice research: training, technology and organisation.

Training

The most important issue is training. Research is a special skill and has its own knowledge that has to be acquired. Bad research is not only a waste of time and money, it is also unethical if it affects patients, and it may well be misleading if it wrongly influences colleagues. In all specialist branches of medicine until recently there has been a formal period of training before doctors became eligible to be appointed as consultants. During this year, which was in effect compulsory in all hospital specialties, doctors were given a day a week of protected time to develop a deep understanding of their specialty and usually to research it. It was common for them to undertake a higher university degree such as a Master's degree or an MD.

General practitioners never had this opportunity because although the Royal College of General Practitioners originally called for a five-year programme of vocational training, including two years in general practice,[13] the reality of vocational training as it was introduced into the UK meant that there was but a single year available for training in general practice itself. This year is fully occupied, indeed crowded, by providing opportunities for young doctors to learn about consultation skills, personal preventive care, and working in homes and families, to say nothing of the increasing complexity of practice management including fund-holding. There simply was never any time to learn about research and although some outstanding trainees did achieve excellent projects, some of which were published in the peer-reviewed literature,[14] these were the exception rather than the rule. The result was that the vast majority of doctors entering general practice did not have competence in doing research and many were left ignorant and suspicious of it. Consequently even the trainers were not able to teach research and over the years a whole education system emerged, including course organisers, GP tutors, associate and regional advisers who had mostly not been trained in, and who were mostly not undertaking research. General practice thus became the only branch of medicine with a twin system of professional leadership: the university departments on the one hand and the directors of postgraduate general practice education (formerly regional advisers) on the other. A number of authors[15–18] have all been urging a more integrated approach, but at the time of writing most registrars (trainees) still do not learn how to do research.

Research skills

There are now many good books available on research in general practice/ primary care and Howie[19] and Carter and Thomas[20] can be recommended. However, it is important that all those who propose doing research or learning to do it have a clear overview about what needs to be learnt.

The first issue is logical thinking and the need to be able to classify and categorise information, to separate ideas and information clearly, and to be able to think deeply about whatever question is being studied. Second, the formulation of an appropriate research question lies at the heart of deciding what is good and bad in research. Most people think that having research ideas is the difficult part but it usually is not. Most GPs can produce a good set of possible ideas. Much harder is the construction of a precise research question, which is capable of being answered to a good level of scientific reliability within the timescale and resources that are available. It often surprises those registering for research degrees to find that it may take many weeks and several supervisions before a research question can be defined and agreed.

The core business of undertaking research is the gathering of information, and the process of data collection is often arduous, frequently frustrating and usually associated with some unexpected problems in obtaining information or in the categories chosen. Data processing used to be a lengthy and laborious part of research but has become relatively easier with the advent of computers and software packages.

A new problem is that primary care workers sometimes rush into research without taking the necessary methodological advice, and particularly statistical advice, which remains just as important as before computers were invented. The final stage is the drawing of conclusions from the data and this requires an open mind, an objective approach and intellectual honesty.

Finally, there is a need to write up the results in a report or paper in a language and style which is acceptable to the editors of peer-reviewed journals and can then be published and used as another building block by the scientific community. Primary care staff have a long-standing deficit in writing skills and unfortunately much interesting research has not always been followed through and written up and published. The old aphorism that unpublished research is failed research is unpopular but true.

The peer-reviewed literature

There are two kinds of journal and the difference between them was most clearly set out by Sir Theodore Fox, who described them as journals of information and journals of record. Both are important and both have a major part to play in the development of the profession and primary care. Journals of information are concerned with the dissemination of information. They typically consist of review or summary articles where someone has worked through a large number of research reports and summarised or abstracted their main findings to make the practical implications and applications possible and practical. Journals of information include journals like *Update*, the medical newspapers and the various bulletins like *Drug and Therapeutics Bulletin, Prescriber's Journal*, etc. They are indispensable tools for all busy clinicians.

Journals of record, however, are different. They are primarily concerned with reporting original research in their particular field. Their priority is simply selecting, in a highly competitive field, the most important research findings which will advance knowledge in the field.

Primary care has a serious shortage of research journals. The first was the then *Journal of the College of General Practitioners*, which was recognised internationally and included in *Index Medicus* in 1961, and is now the *British Journal of General Practice*.[21] *Index Medicus*, however, only includes 11 journals or equivalent and it is a tribute to the academic community in primary care in the UK that five of these are published in the UK. It is also encouraging that the highest-ranked peer-reviewed journal in general practice/primary care worldwide is the *British Journal of General Practice*. Its international impact factor of 2.29 places it 12th out of 115 general medical journals in the world.[22] It is not only the highest-ranked primary care journal worldwide but it is the only clinical specialty in which the UK has the highest-ranked journal. It is published by a British organisation, the Royal College of General Practitioners, and in 1998, it is edited by a British GP, Alastair Wright.

The price of this success, however, is high, and currently about 90% of articles submitted to that journal are rejected. Hence there is a serious shortage of space for peer-reviewed publications and it is a matter of increasing concern that primary care is still inadequately catered for in this respect.

Research qualifications

In addition to the basic qualifications in medicine, the university world has, over the years, developed a number of degrees specifically concerned with research, which is a core function for universities. Indeed universities are the only organisations in our society which are specifically charged with the responsibility of doing research and in which research expertise is demanded for staff appointments.

These degrees sometimes cause confusion but are not difficult to understand. At Bachelor's level, the BSc, most commonly undertaken by medical students on an intercalated basis, has for many years provided a basic grounding in research methods. It is interesting that many of those now active in research in general practice have previously undertaken a BSc.

At the Master's level the commonest degree is MSc and in most universities this is a taught degree, i.e. the postgraduate students attend a formal course and although they are naturally expected to undertake a good deal of work on their own, the programme of learning is essentially taught.

A number of universities, however, offer an alternative route to a Masters degree through an MPhil by research. This is a research degree and is based on 2–4 years of research. These degrees have proved attractive to primary care staff and a growing number of GPs, practice nurses and members of the professions allied to medicine are now acquiring them. They can be warmly recommended as a practical and feasible way of learning about research, actually doing research appropriate to primary care and obtaining an internationally recognised research qualification.

At the highest university level there are two degrees. The PhD normally requires registering for three years full time or equivalent part time, and this has limited the possibilities for working GPs, although about a dozen have succeeded since the Second World War. An alternative route to a doctoral degree is the MD. This is the gold standard for research in general practice but it too has had a chequered career for GPs, mainly because of lack of skills and sustained support, often over many years. The Royal College of General Practitioners and the university departments of general practice are vigorously encouraging GPs to do MDs and it is encouraging that an increasing number are succeeding. In any one year about a dozen GPs now obtain an MD from one or other of the medical schools in the UK. A higher degree is now a prerequisite for appointment to the academic staff of most universities and those who hope to become lecturers, senior lecturers or professors should now assume this and obtain the necessary qualifications as early in their professional careers as possible.

Technology

A second major obstacle to undertaking research in general practice has been the problem of handling a huge amount of information. Specialist medicine has the ability to focus down and has advanced by focusing its research effort on smaller and smaller fields in which it has been consistently successful. However, generalist medicine can only focus down on a narrow research question at a price. It inevitably has to do so, because the research method demands focus. Nevertheless, the danger of a narrow approach is that some of the essence of general practice as a human and psychosocial discipline gets lost. The advent of computers has made a major difference. Starting with the 'Micros for GPs' scheme, sponsored by the Department of Health in 1983,[23] and aided by some commercial developments, primary-care computing has developed so swiftly that by the late 1990s British GPs were using desktop computers more than GPs in other Western countries, and very much more than NHS consultants in the hospital service.

Although the time involved, both for doctors and staff, in inputting large amounts of medical, psychological and social information has been immense, and is still continuing, the stage has been reached, as the end of the century approaches, when primary-care clinical databases are among the most accurate and comprehensive in the NHS, and indeed in Europe. The stage is therefore set for general practice to harness its own clinical information for the purposes of research for the first time ever.

Organisation

The third obstacle has been the organisational characteristics of general practice. When the Royal College of General Practitioners was founded about 40% of GPs were singlehanded and a substantial majority were in one- or two-partner practices. The progressive development of good practice and the multiprofessional primary healthcare team has not only brought a wider range of skills but division of labour and in particular the introduction of computer operators, who are in some practices now developing into research assistants.

Finally, in 1994, the idea of the funded research general practice was reintroduced, funded first by the Royal College of General Practitioners from subscription income. This idea was, as had originally been hoped, picked up by the NHS, so that NHS-funded research and development practices have now been approved in England, Scotland and Wales. Indeed the NHS Executive has now committed to this initiative over £1 million.

Clearly, however, research in general practice can never wholly depend, nor should it depend, on single research practices – however successful. Some of the research questions in primary care require a population which is too great for any one general practice to have enough patients to give the necessary power to answer the question at all.[24] There is therefore a need to group research active practices. Here, the huge contribution of the university departments of general practice has become clear and they have, with the Birmingham Research Unit and the Manchester Research Unit of the Royal College of General Practitioners, been the main organisations which have undertaken research across general practices over the years.

The crucial idea of categorising patients by age and sex was first put forward by Watts[25] and vigorously promulgated by the Royal College of General Practitioners' Birmingham Unit. It was the Birmingham Unit that disseminated ideas like the morbidity register or E book, which had been introduced by Eimerl.[26]

The university departments of general practice have grown steadily in numbers and resources as well as influence. At the time of writing (October 1998) there were departments of general practice in every medical school,[27] and there are now 50 professors of general practice or of general practice/primary care in the UK.

The latest development, fostered particularly by exciting initiatives in the Northern Region,[28] Trent[29] and Wessex (WReN personal communication 1997), has been the development of primary care research networks funded by the NHS. These networks are, by and large, constructed to encourage and support working doctors and nurses in primary care to enable them to develop their own research ideas and to introduce a greatly enhanced attitude to research through increased research skills and competence in primary care. To do this it has been necessary to harness the academic experience of research, which in general practice lies mainly in the university departments. In most primary care research networks, one or more university departments of general practice are actively involved. The intention is thus to link research expertise with research opportunity.

In December 1996, the Secretary of State for Health, in the third of the 1996 White Papers, issued a commitment to foster primary care research networks and to double the spending on primary care research in the following five years.[30]

THE FUTURE

Research in general practice/primary care stands at a crossroads. It has passed the end of the development stage and has now achieved entry to all the medical schools and a core of professors. However, much research in general practice has been disappointing and indeed Marinker[31] once said that most research from university departments of general practice has either simply confirmed the expected or has been banal. There are organisational as well as academic reasons for this and the university departments have been under pressure within their universities to prove themselves. They have often been driven by external funding pressures or relationships within the medical schools to research on topics that were not always absolutely core to general practice as a discipline.

However, with the advent of government policy to develop a primary care-led NHS[32] the time has probably now come when multiprofessional departments of general practice/primary care can increasingly seek to research the core issues of general practice/family medicine which are in urgent need of study and which make general practice special among all the other branches of medical practice. Pereira Gray[33] speaking at the *Referatentag* of the universities of general practice in the Netherlands suggested eight key features or priorities, which would guide the research strategy for general practice research in the future and these were:

- primary assessment
- a family perspective
- a domiciliary perspective at least in Europe
- continuity of care
- personal preventive medicine
- relationship with a person as a whole human being (holistic care)
- caring for a defined population of registered patients
- understanding of the resources available and a commitment to their most efficient use.

CONCLUSION

The conclusion is, therefore, that general practice as a profession has become academically fragmented, with the university departments too separate from the directors of postgraduate general practice education, and a serious deficiency in research skills permeates primary care.

The main source of research in general practice/primary care is the university departments of general practice/primary care. However, they are having to work hard to maintain and develop their departments within a university world beset by funding problems and in which new groupings are occurring which are likely to be much bigger and in which identity for general practice/primary care will be harder to maintain.

The new organisational groupings, especially the RCGP and NHS research general practices and the NHS research networks, can be expected to do much to counter this fragmentation. They will bring colleagues together, and change the research culture in primary care through showing the potential for and the achievement of substantial success in research in primary care.

General practice research has a bright future, with more people interested in it than before and with a greater number and therefore proportion of research active colleagues than ever before. There is a steadily increasing number of GPs who hold university qualifications at masters or doctoral level. The power of computing, the rising number in the primary healthcare team and the growing government attention towards primary care all give grounds for optimism. For the minority of colleagues who find research intellectually fascinating and professionally rewarding, the future is bright.

REFERENCES

1. Budd W (1873) *Typhoid Fever.* Longmans Green, London.

2. Mackenzie J (1916) *Principles of Diagnosis and Treatment in Heart Affections.* Henry Frowde, London.

3. Pickles WN (1939) *Epidemiology and Country Practice.* John Wright, Bristol. Republished by Royal College of General Practitioners, London.

4. Crombie DL (1963) The defects of general practice. *Lancet.* **1**: 209–11.

5. Fry J (1977) Commonsense and uncommon sensibility. James MacKenzie Lecture 1976. *Journal of the Royal College of General Practitioners.* **27**: 9–17.

6. Tudor Hart J (1980) *Hypertension.* Churchill Livingstone, Edinburgh.

7. Stott NCH and West RR (1976) Randomised controlled trial of antibiotics in patients with cough and purulent sputum. *BMJ.* **2**: 556–9.

8. Kinmonth A-L, Angus RM and Baum JD (1982) Whole food and increased dietary fibre improve blood glucose control in diabetic children. *Archives of Disease in Childhood.* **57**: 187–94.

9. Howie JGR, Heaney DJ and Maxwell M (1997) *Measuring Quality in General Practice.* Occasional Paper 75. Royal College of General Practitioners, Exeter.

10. Office of Population Censuses and Surveys (1991) *General Household Survey.* HMSO, London.

11. Pereira Gray D (1995) Primary care and the public health. Harben Lecture 1994. *Health and Hygiene.* **16**: 49–62.

12. Pereira Gray D (1991) Research in general practice: law of inverse opportunity. *BMJ.* **302**: 1380–2.

13. College of General Practitioners (1965*) Special Vocational Training for General Practice. Report from General Practice 1.* CGP, London.

14. Trainee Syntex Award Winners 1981–1984 (1985) *Trainee Projects.* Occasional Paper 29. Royal College of General Practitioners, London.

15. Allen J, Wilson A, Fraser R *et al.* (1993) The academic base for general practice: the case for change. *BMJ.* **307**: 719–22.

16. Pereira Gray D (1993) Two sides of the coin. *Postgraduate Education for General Practice.* **4**: 85–8.

17. Hannay D (1994) Undergraduate and postgraduate medical education: bridging the divide. Editorial. *British Journal of General Practice.* **44**: 487–8.

18. Rashid A, Allen J, Styles W *et al.* (1994) Careers in academic general practice: constraints and opportunities. *BMJ.* **309**: 1270–2.

19. Howie JGR (1979) *Research in General Practice.* Croom Helm, London.

20. Carter Y and Thomas C (1997) *Research Methods in Primary Care.* Radcliffe Medical Press, Oxford.

21. Pereira Gray D (1989) The emergence of the discipline of general practice, its literature and the contribution of the College *Journal.* McConaghey Memorial Lecture 1988. *Journal of the Royal College of General Practitioners.* **39**: 228–33.

22. Institute for Scientific Information (1996) *Science Citation Index.* ISI, Philadelphia, USA.

23. DHSS and the Joint Computer Policy Group (1985) *Micros in Practice.* Report of an Appraisal of GP Microcomputer Systems. HMSO, London.

24. Campbell MJ, Julious SA and Altman DG (1995) Estimating sample size for binary, ordered categorical and continuous outcomes in two group comparisons. *BMJ.* **311**: 1145–8.

25. Watts CAH (1958) How to compile an age–sex register. *Between Ourselves.* No. 8, 1–12.

26. Eimerl TS (1960) Organized curiosity. A practical approach to the problem of keeping records for research purposes in general practice. *Journal of the College of General Practitioners.* **3**: 246–52.

27. Connection (1996) Professors of General Practice/Primary Care and GPs who hold professorial posts in the UK and Ireland. *British Journal of General Practice.* **46**: viii.

28. Northern Primary Care Research Network (1996) *NoReN Report 1995–96.* NoReN, Stockton-on-Tees.

29. Trent Focus (1997) *Annual Report.* University of Nottingham, Nottingham.

30. Secretary of State for Health (1996) *Primary Care – delivering the future.* Cm 3512. The Stationery Office, London, para 3.19.

31. Marinker M (1994) *The End of General Practice*. Eighth Bayliss Lecture. HMSO, London.

32. Dorrell S (1996) *Primary Care: the Future*. NHS Executive, Leeds.

33. Pereira Gray D (1996) Research in general practice. *European Journal of General Practice*. **2**: 126–8.

2

Research networks

Pali Hungin

The era of primary care research networks in the UK was heralded by the Northern Primary Care Research Network (NoReN) and the Wessex Primary Care Research Network (WReN) in the early 1990s. Unusually for British general practice this followed a much longer tradition from the USA, where the Ambulatory Sentinel Practice Network (ASPN) was, amongst others, an established network of some years standing for data pooling and research facilitation. Over the last five years, primary care networks have emerged in most parts of the UK and are now considered an integral part of research and development nationally.[1] Prominent networks in the UK now include the South Thames Research and Implementation Network (STaRNet), the Trent Focus and the Midlands Research Network (MidReN).

The development of networks in the UK has been a response to the inherent problems afflicting research in primary care, and particularly general practice, which is the largest portion of primary care. Although opinion is now swinging in favour of recognising the potential of research from primary care and the aspirations of practice-based researchers, many of the handicaps identified during the last decade remain.[2] These include:

- the lack of an established research culture in general practice
- the lack of opportunity for research, particularly protected time
- lack of training and easy access to experts and resources.

The early networks have contributed to the reassessment of the role of primary care professionals in research, and, with the newer ones, now provide structures through which change can be effected. Together with the departments of general practice in the universities, many of which have been relatively handicapped in this regard because of a heavy undergraduate teaching load, research networks offer the tantalising possibility of engaging with primary care in a practical manner.

A challenge for practice-based research is the requirement to maintain the highest standards. The markers of quality include the following:

- Rigour at all stages, especially when formulating research questions and methodologies.

- Ensuring reproducibility and generalisability of the research, factors often dependent on appropriate sampling and numbers. This has been a problem for the lone researcher in general practice.
- Using meaningful expert input at all stages, especially during planning.
- A need for the research to remain responsive to the real questions and the development requirements in healthcare.

MODELS OF NETWORKS

Broadly, networks have been referred to as either being organised on (i) a 'top-down' basis, where the initiative is usually led from an academic institution or (ii) a 'bottom-up' basis, where the leadership and organisation is service-practitioner led. In reality, nearly all UK networks are based on partnership between academic centres and practitioners, while encompassing wide variations in style and structure dependent on how the initiative started. Some networks, e.g. STaRNet, are groupings of remunerated research practices, centrally coordinated for research training, mentoring and collaborative research, while others, such as NoReN and WReN, are a mix of a practitioner-based cooperative with designated research practices.[3]

THE NoReN EXPERIENCE

NoReN was established in 1991 as the result of collaboration between the Royal College of General Practitioners, the University of Newcastle upon Tyne and the Northern Regional Health Authority. It follows the 'bottom-up' model and was set up as a multidisciplinary cooperative of primary care practitioners in northern England, in conjunction with the university department of primary care. It is an independent organisation, without formal ties with an outside body, and the director reports directly to the Northern and Yorkshire NHS Executive. During 1997, 12 remunerated research practices were appointed within the NoReN locality and will be supported by NoReN. NoReN's multidisciplinary steering group is drawn from its membership and consists mainly of practice-based individuals and academics from local universities.

Guiding principles

1. Investing in people. Recognising that meaningful change is effected by motivated individuals and not systems alone.
2. Creating an environment in which research is seen as a positive attribute and a necessity for the development of the profession.

3. Preparing a structured support system for fostering research.
4. Developing an education and career structure for practice-based researchers, including attachments and appointments, and help towards higher degrees and diplomas.
5. Being part of an integrated drive towards research and development and to ensure representation for primary care researchers at policy making and resource allocation level.

Membership

NoReN activities and facilities are open to anyone linked with health and are advertised regionwide. Formal membership is through an annual subscription which enables attendance at educational events at reduced cost and provides an active mailing list for specific communications. Members have diverse backgrounds, with GPs comprising 50% of the total. The membership includes district nurses, practice nurses, health visitors, speech therapists, physiotherapists, counsellors and staff from audit groups.

Funding and staff

Funding is provided by the Northern and Yorkshire NHS Executive, mainly from its Budget 2 category of research and development funds, for (i) basic infrastructure, including office and staff costs, and (ii) research training activities. The research practices, while supported by NoReN, are funded directly by the Executive. Some additional funding is available from subscriptions, nominal fees for educational events and from service costs from collaborative research. Staff consists of a part-time manager, a full-time secretary, a part-time research coordinator, a part-time liaison practitioner and a part-time remunerated GP director. NoReN also has two part-time research fellows funded by a non-recurring grant to the University of Newcastle upon Tyne.

Activities

NoReN's activities are geared towards research training, mentoring and fostering collaborative research. Specific activities during 1997 included the following:

- A research training programme, typically of 8–12 one-day or half-day events, evening classes and a major national research conference.
- Personal mentoring to researchers on a one-to-one basis.
- Open-access research counselling from contacts within the network and NoReN staff.

- Facilitating special interest groups, e.g. on women's health, gastroenterology and prescribing.
- Coordinating collaborative research, e.g. projects requiring large-scale practitioner participation.
- Holding an annual research presentation day as a showcase event for local research.
- Providing an interface with other local groups, e.g. hospital research committees.
- Representing primary care researchers at policy making and executive level within the regional research and development programme.

Assessing success

This is a thorny problem for networks, most of whom see their remit as facilitation and nurturing rather than as academic foci for research output. The traditional criteria for assessing academic success by publications, research awards and higher degrees can be difficult for networks to demonstrate, especially in the early years. Indeed, the role of networks contributing to such success can be difficult to evaluate if the successful individuals have other affiliations. Nonetheless, within the NoReN locality there has been a demonstrable increase in practice-based research in association with a steady stream of publications and grant successes.

A particular success of the networking process has been an increase in the level of collaboration between different academic centres and a reduction of traditional academic barriers. NoReN linked grant applications now commonly include participation from experts from several institutions, encompassing different skills. Equally importantly, by providing a recognisable interface for those outside primary care, NoReN members have profited from opportunities for meaningful collaboration with others in different settings. Perhaps most notably, networks have an important role in reversing the decline of the research culture in primary care and there are indications that practice-based researchers in the north of England are rediscovering confidence and research success.

STaRNet: South Thames Research and Implementation Network of general practices

Tony Kendrick

A new research network in South Thames: starting from scratch

The vision behind STaRNet came from a growing recognition that the research base of general practice needed strengthening to support the development of the primary care-led NHS. The plan to establish the network drew, to an extent, on the experience of GPs in other networks, notably the national MRC GP Research Framework, NoReN in the Northern and Yorkshire Region and WReN in Wessex. However, the method of recruitment and expansion of the network was unique.

In 1996, a joint proposal for funding a new network of research and development general practices was put to the regional R&D directorate by the three heads of departments of general practice in South Thames, Professors Sean Hilton (St George's), Roger Jones (UMDS) and Roger Higgs (King's), in collaboration with the two postgraduate deans of general practice education, Drs Ri Hornung and Alan Ruben. The directorate awarded a grant of around £880 000 to fund the setting up of the network in the first two years. This included a sum of £10 000 per annum for each of the first 15 member practices ('lead practices') as well as funding for research training costs and the salaries of the project team of seven research staff based in the three medical schools, supported by a network administrator at St George's. The direction of the project is overseen by a steering group which meets quarterly at the NHS Executive South Thames.

The aims of STaRNet

The initial development of STaRNet therefore was 'top-down', i.e. led by senior academics with generous funding from the regional R&D directorate. This may be contrasted with the development of NoReN, which was led by an ever-burgeoning group of practitioners who were interested in research and decided to get together in a 'bottom-up' fashion and attract resources to help them.

Box 2.1 Aims of STaRNet

- To develop a framework for multipractice research by means of contracting with a number of research and development practices (initially 15 lead practices)
- To develop primary care-led research through training, support and assistance in project development
- To provide a network for dissemination of information, evidence-based practice and clinical guidelines, and to assess the impact of these on health outcomes
- To assist the 15 lead research and development practices in setting up local groupings of associate practices with interests in research, critical appraisal and evidence-based practice

---

The aims of STaRNet were clearly laid out in the original submission for funding, and are listed in Box 2.1.

Recruitment of the 15 lead R&D practices

The first 15 'lead practices' were recruited through adverts placed in the *BMJ* and sent through the health authorities' mailing system to all South Thames practices. Initial applications were received from 86 practices, which is 9% of the total in the region. Thirty practices were shortlisted for interview and 15 selected on the basis of their keenness, research and audit experience, practice organisation and geographical location (to ensure a spread across the region).

Initial needs assessment

After recruitment, an assessment of needs for training in research methods and evidence-based practice was carried out among the lead GPs and other interested health professionals within the practices.

Teaching course

An initial teaching course in research methods and evidence-based healthcare was then designed to enable the 15 lead GPs, together with a second interested member of each lead practice, to initiate a research project within their own practice or together with other practices, and to evaluate the research literature critically. The course consisted of 13 half-day sessions.

Resource packs on research methods and evidence-based practice

At the first STaRNet teaching session a research methods resource pack was distributed to each lead practice. This was developed by the STaRNet project team, and included information, references and key articles on: literature reviewing, questionnaires and surveys, qualitative research, epidemiology, clinical trials, evaluating healthcare, health economics research, statistics, ethical issues, writing up and disseminating research, applying for funding and using the Internet in research. A second resource pack was developed on evidence-based healthcare to support the STaRNet lead practices in their work on implementing clinical guidelines and developing evidence-based practice. The pack provided references to key publications and detailed information about groups and resources concerned with evidence-based healthcare and included sections on: an overview of the evidence-based healthcare movement, how to find research evidence, critical appraisal, systematic reviews, guidelines, audit and managing change.

Practices' own research projects

Although the recruitment and initial training of network practices was 'top-down', all the member practices were encouraged to develop their own ideas for research projects within the first year after recruitment. Members of the STaRNet project team provide development support through meetings to discuss, support, advise and give feedback on practices' projects. Some projects were relatively small and limited to within one lead practice. Others involved their associate practices in multipractice studies. Where appropriate, practices were encouraged and assisted to draw up grant applications to other funding bodies.

Projects being developed within the lead practices included: a randomised controlled trial of nurse versus doctor management of common acute minor problems in general practice, the impact on practice activity of mental health workers in general practices and differences in GPs' behaviour with regard to follow-up appointments.

STaRNet group of research projects

Members of the 15 lead practices also agreed that at least one STaRNet group research project should commence in the first year after recruitment. Possible ideas concerned: problems arising from earlier hospital discharge, provision of contraceptive services by practice nurses, use of normal ranges for peak flow, treatment of osteoporosis following fractures and oral steroid prescriptions in asthma.

Research projects conducted by outside organisations through STaRNet

Any proposals received for possible research projects funded and conducted by outside organisations must be presented to the STaRNet steering group for consideration. Such proposals would need to include payments to cover any proposed involvement of members of the STaRNet project team and of the participating practices. If so funded, members of the project team might discuss and if necessary modify any such projects together with the outside organisation and with the practices within STaRNet that might potentially be involved in such research. Participation by practices in any such projects would be entirely voluntary. A written policy has been developed by the steering group for dealing with approaches to STaRNet from outside bodies wishing to use the network for research projects.

Implementation of evidence-based healthcare

Each of the 15 lead practices implemented one clinical guideline in their practice, and will be helped to audit the outcome of such implementation in due course. The STaRNet coordinating team offered the 15 lead practices a choice of one out of four evidence-based cardiovascular guidelines, listed in Box 2.2.

Box 2.2 Cardiovascular evidence-based guidelines implemented in STaRNet

- Aspirin and beta-blocker use post-myocardial infarction
- ACE inhibitors in heart failure
- Management of hypertension in the elderly
- Use of cholesterol-lowering drugs

These guidelines were presented to the lead practices by the STaRNet team within the first month after recruitment of the practices. Where possible, practices were asked to involve their local associate practices in the implementation of the guidelines. The lead practices were encouraged to make minor modifications to the guidelines where necessary to suit their particular practices and the way they function. Lead practices are also being encouraged to take up and develop other evidence-based guidelines of their own, in other clinical areas. This will involve searching and critically appraising the literature (including meta-analyses and systematic reviews), requesting a specialist expert opinion where necessary, reaching a consensus within the practice and producing a written protocol. It is hoped that guidelines would also involve other local associate practices where possible.

Activities of the associate practices

Each of the 15 lead practices was asked to identify and recruit at least five associate practices within the first six months of the project, encouraged and supported in this recruitment by the coordinating medical schools. The aims of recruiting associate practices were to develop a culture of primary care research and implementation of evidence-based healthcare throughout a network of practices beyond the initial 15 lead practices, and eventually for associate practices to participate in research and implementation projects led by the lead practices locally, or in multipractice studies coordinated centrally by the medical schools. Associate membership is open to individuals as well as to whole practices.

Evaluation of STaRNet

The ongoing evaluation of STaRNet includes measures of structure, process and outcome. Structural measures included those listed in Box 2.3. Process measures include those listed in Box 2.4.

Box 2.3   Structural measures
- Numbers of associate practices recruited
- Numbers of GPs and other professionals taking an active part in the network, including attendance at training courses and meetings
- IT links in place between the practices and each other, and between the practices and the supporting medical school departments

---

Box 2.4   Process measures

- Changes in confidence, and reported behaviours among member GPs and other professionals, measured using the questionnaires administered before, and repeated after, the training in research methods and evidence-based healthcare
- Interview and questionnaire measures of professionals' satisfaction with the training received
- Numbers of proposals submitted for funding
- Numbers of research projects in progress led by member practices, and other research projects being conducted through STaRNet
- Research papers submitted for publication, or presented at conferences
- Numbers of guidelines implemented
- Changes in the process of patient care including diagnostic tests, treatment and follow up, assessed by examining patient records before and after implementation

---

General practice research networks: a user's view

Michael Moore and Felicity Thompson

How we became interested

In 1993, I had been a full-time GP in a service general practice for 5 years. I had undertaken some research both as an undergraduate and postgraduate, but my single attempt at general practice research remained dusty, unpublished and unpublishable. Nevertheless, I harboured a desire to broaden my horizons and develop my interest in research. I signed up at short notice for a research methods course held in the local academic department of general practice. Following this stimulating course my cover was blown and I was recruited into the fledgling Wessex Research Network (WReN). One of our practice nurses (FT) has since also become involved in research. The following describes how our membership of a research network has had an impact on our lives both at work and at home.

The research network

The WReN began life in 1994 as a collaborative venture between the Royal College of General Practitioners, Southampton University Department of Primary Care and the Wessex Regional Health Authority (now South and Western Regional Health Authority). The network has six major objectives:

- developing a network organisation and infrastructure
- identifying primary healthcare teams interested in R&D
- providing individual research support
- supporting the development of network projects
- promoting research awareness, knowledge and skills in primary care
- enabling appropriate research with others.

Two key barriers to research in primary care had been identified by the research subcommittee of the local College faculty, namely the lack of protected time and lack of research skills. The network has endeavoured to overcome these barriers through the innovative bursary scheme. Financial assistance is available to the primary healthcare team. Members are encouraged to apply for funding to allow them time to identify research questions, undertake a literature review, meet with experts, complete funding applications and write up completed research. The WReN directorate takes an active role in research support providing expert advice free of charge to its members.

The network has primarily taken a 'bottom-up' approach to encouraging primary care research activity. Members are encouraged to participate in research methods courses and then to pursue their own research agenda. More recently, network projects have been developed by the steering group to utilise the power inherent within the network.

Membership of the network is free and open to all members of the primary healthcare team. New members are encouraged to provide information about their educational needs and their areas of research interest. At its basic level, membership of the network may simply involve the practice in receipt of the quarterly newsletter and occasional invitations to participate or collaborate in research activities. Information provided by the members enables identification of members with particular interests, and targeting of approaches is possible.

What we have achieved

Our own involvement has grown rapidly from simple membership. Through the network newsletter and direct approaches we have identified projects that excite interest within the practice and we have participated in a number of network projects (identification of preventable risk factors post-myocardial infarction, survey of asthma leaflets) and projects originating outside the network (use of information leaflets in repeat pill users). My first project arose from comments made by network members and was undertaken in collaboration with the network director, Helen Smith. Practices were recruited throughout Wessex using the network to study the volume of research requests received in primary care. This project was funded by the RCGP and is in preparation for publication.

In 1995, we were invited through the WReN network to collaborate with a funded project looking at telephone nurse triage for out-of-hours care. The pilot project was undertaken within the practice and the main randomised controlled trial took place in the local GP cooperative. In the same year, I used a WReN bursary to allow me to prepare a successful application for research infrastructure funding from the South and Western Regional Health Authority. We are now a South and Western Regional Research General Practice. The practice receives funding which allows other clinical team members and me to use protected time for research activity. Since becoming a research practice we have established links with many other organisations and groups. We are involved in a number of collaborative projects and we have made a bid for Culyer funding to continue the work after the three years of South and Western funding.

The effects on the practice

We are a four (now five-) partner practice with a list size of 7000 patients in the cathedral city of Salisbury. The practice is predominantly urban (>90%) and approximates to the national average in terms of age and sex distribution.

The impact on the practice has grown steadily with time. It is difficult to identify where the demands on a network practice are different from the demands on a research general practice, as one state led to another. The practice has to deal with the regular absence of one partner. We coped initially with a retained doctor plus irregular locums. Last year we decided to expand the partnership with an additional half-time partner part-funded through research funding. This strategy, while solving the locum problem, is not without risk to the partnership given the short-term nature of the research funding.

We regularly run up to three trials within the practice and are frequently involved in recruiting patients for trials outside the practice. Additional workload arises both in consultation and in administration for the practice staff. I have to justify to my partners the value of identifying and recruiting patients for clinical trials often without reward when they are hard-pressed in busy surgeries. The staff bear with me when I ask for yet another basket of notes so I can sift through, identifying suitable candidates for outside researchers, while not infrequently they find a researcher camped in a consultation room making further demands on space and time.

As our critical appraisal skills have grown we have adopted a number of evidence-based guidelines and have become more confident in evaluating the evidence for new drugs and procedures. We are more likely to question 'standard practice'. The involvement of the primary healthcare team has aided team development. Both practice nurses, one receptionist and one partner have also been able to attend research methods courses. We have an annual research day when presentations regarding ongoing research are made to the primary health-care team. We have established regular meetings with another local research practice hopefully as a prelude to establishing a local research interest group.

Effect on patients

There are the obvious effects of carrying the trial burden in that the patients are more likely to be asked to consent to participation in a randomised clinical trial. There are less obvious positive benefits derived from our greater awareness of research findings and greater willingness to implement them. These range from our use of evidence-based patient care protocols to our unwillingness to purchase treatments which have not been shown to be effective. Participation in clinical trials raises the awareness of the conditions under study and makes us more critical of accepted practice.

The effect on personal development

The doctor's view

There has been a substantial effect on my professional and personal life, both positive and negative. I have found my involvement in research both stimulating and enjoyable. I established contacts and friendships with a wide variety of people outside primary care. My reduced clinical commitment has paradoxically led to increased enjoyment; I no longer dread the Monday morning surgery because on Wednesday I am considering unanswered questions as potential research material. I feel in control of my situation and have greater self-confidence as a result of increased awareness of the current literature.

There are two main disadvantages. First, it is difficult to maintain continuity of care with regular absence from practice, the patients like to see *their* doctor any day of the week. Second, as I remain a full-time partner I retain a high clinical and administrative workload, all of which is sandwiched into a shrinking working week. I more often stay late to complete leftover work, I attend more evening meetings and often work late at home. Despite working less clinical time my overall workload has increased. On the positive side, some days I work from home and even manage to join the family for an evening meal. I feel that my research work has made me a happier person.

The nurse's view

Practice nursing was an ideal return from a 'childcare retirement' for me. Part-time hours in a friendly and innovative surgery was a perfect environment to acquire and learn experientially the new skills and knowledge required to update my training. My nurse teaching background helped to integrate theory and practice and the inevitable self-managed workload. Many of my existing skills were utilised in writing practice protocols and guidelines for all members of the multidisciplinary team to follow.

Primary care research activity mainly functioned around medical models, but the local audit programme and the doctors encouraged me to examine and evaluate areas of nursing practice and care, e.g. travel vaccinations, cold chain vaccine storage and phlebotomy services. In essence, I was beginning to use an evidence base to look critically at areas of nursing care and differentiate good and bad working patterns.

Two major stimuli into research activity were having Mike as an enthusiastic innovator at the practice with supportive partners and undertaking the research methods course held by the WReN network. These enabled me to gain insight into a multidisciplinary approach to research with a sound knowledge base to utilise in projects and trials associated with the local research network.

Networking and establishing links have led to collaboration with researchers from the University of Southampton to set up a randomised controlled trial of out-of-hours nurse telephone triage. This has encouraged me to act as an innovator in nurse practice and allow my own practice to be assessed and evaluated, thus helping to develop, mould and guide future nursing practice.

Working with other research personnel has widened the boundaries of my role. It has allowed me to network with other nurses and members of a multidisciplinary team to build on my existing knowledge and to search for new information and evidence on which to base practice. Many of the new skills extrapolated from the research involvement have been fully utilised. One such important new skill has been the ability to search for relevant nursing and medical literature and critically appraise and analyse the information.

Encouragement from the practice and research team has given me confidence to begin to write for publication and to present papers at study days and conferences. This has enabled me to travel and disseminate my area of practice with others doing similar projects and work.

One problem of becoming involved in research is the change in work environment and practice. Inevitably this unsettles the working teams in the surgery, making it essential to keep communication channels open and regularly update everyone with new plans and practice. Time is always a limiting factor. Clinical work and patient care always seem to erode into those research meetings and the family also seem to need attention and care at times too. Hobbies seem to be on hold, but maybe research is becoming one! Enthusiasm, dedication and determination to achieve would be very high on my list of research priorities.

However, I have found that research has been exciting, fulfilling and at times frustrating, but very worthwhile. It has opened up future pathways for my career development and allowed me to help realise my potential. Using my new skills and knowledge I am hoping to undertake a Masters programme in research methods which will help develop the processes of care within practice nursing and primary care.

We have great hopes for the future. We have submitted a bid for Culyer funding in order to continue to support the research activity within our team. We have established a multidisciplinary network of contacts. We feel that as a service general practice we have some real value to offer the academic community both in terms of framing relevant research questions and understanding what is feasible within primary care.

Box 2.5   Key points
- Greater job satisfaction
- Strengthens primary healthcare team
- Improved critical reading skills leads to better use of available evidence
- Increased workload
- Service general practices have valuable role in framing relevant, achievable and do-able research questions

---

REFERENCES

1. Secretary of State for Health (1996) *Primary Care: the future*. NHS Executive, London.

2. Royal College of General Practitioners (1990) *The 1990 Report of the Research Task Force*. RCGP, London.

3. Evans D, Exworthy M, Peckham S *et al.* (1997) *Primary Care Research Networks: report to the NHS Executive South and West*. Institute for Health Policy Studies, University of Southampton.

FURTHER READING

Beasley J (1993) The structure and activity of Primary Care Research Networks. *Family Research Journal*. **13**: 395–6.

Department of Health (1997) *NHS Funding for Research and Development*. DoH, London.

Department of Health (1997) *Report of the Working Party on Research and Development in Primary Care. The Mant Report*. DoH, London.

Haines A and Jones R (1994) Implementing findings of research. *BMJ*. **308**: 1488–92.

Howie JGR (1988) *Report of the Working Group on Research in Health Care in the Community.* Scottish Home and Health Department, Edinburgh.

Howie JGR (1996) Addressing the credibility gap in general practice research: better theory, more feeling, less strategy. *British Journal of General Practice.* **46**: 479–81.

Hungin APS (1995) *Research Networks in Primary Care in the UK: a national report.* Northern Primary Care Research Network (NoReN), Stockton on Tees.

Jones R (1990) International family practice research. *Family Practice.* **7**: 2.

Pereira Gray D (1991) Research in general practice: law of inverse opportunity. *BMJ*. **302**: 1380–2.

Pereira Gray D (1996) Research general practices. *British Journal of General Practice.* **45**: 516–17.

Williams WO (1990) A survey of doctorates by thesis among general practitioners in the British Isles from 1973 to 1988. *British Journal of General Practice.* **40**: 491–4.

3

The MRC General Practice Research Framework

Background, research and organisation

Madge Vickers

The Medical Research Council (MRC) General Practice Research Framework (GPRF) is an organisation of around 900 general practices throughout the UK involved in epidemiological and health services research. The activities of the GPRF are coordinated by the MRC Epidemiology and Medical Care Unit (EMCU).

HISTORY

From the beginning the GPRF has been project led. It was originally set up in the early 1970s by Dr Bill Miall (EMCU) for the MRC mild hypertension trial. Three approaches to recruiting clinics for the pilot trial were tried, screening organisations, large industrial companies and general practices, and the expectation was that the first two would be more successful. Bill Miall recalls, however, that he 'had quite mistakenly doubted the willingness and ability of busy GPs to embark on blood pressure screening programmes and to follow a complicated protocol designed by a committee of so-called hypertension "experts" who had little or no experience of general practice'. The full-scale trial eventually involved 190 clinics of which 176 were general practices. The GPRF was born.

The mild hypertension trial lasted 12 years from pilot to publication and all the practices completed the trial. Long before the end of the trial Bill Miall realised that the group of practices he had set up provided 'a valuable facility for epidemiological research into other common diseases or for research into general practice itself'. Professor Sir Stanley Peart, the chairman of the trial working party, went further, expressing the view that 'the demonstration that a team of busy general practitioners could successfully carry out a research project of this size and complexity was more important than demonstrating whether or not it was of value to treat people with mild hypertension'. The reader must decide whether he was right.

Bill Miall's starting point for recruitment was a list of practices from the Royal College of General Practitioners, supplemented later by practices responding to an advertisement in the *BMJ* and other journals and by personal recommendation from existing members. His approach was as follows:

• letter to the practice summarising plans and how MRC could help
• personal lunchtime visit to the practice to meet all partners, practice nurses and the practice manager
• follow-up visit by a training nurse
• full training in the study for the nurses and GPs involved in the trial.

Visiting the practices was time-consuming but invaluable in assessing the enthusiasm of all practice staff and ensuring that there was adequate space for trial work. Half the practices visited joined the trial, about one quarter were judged unsuitable, often because one or more partners were unsure about participating, and the rest decided not to join.

From the practice viewpoint the gains were:

• contributing to answering an important medical question
• computerisation of age–sex registers when this was a rarity
• reimbursement of nurse time for trial work
• sessional fees for GP involvement
• training for nurses and GPs in trial procedures.

When the second hypertension trial in older patients started in 1981, the GPRF was expanded to around 250 practices. Bill Miall retired in 1983. Dr Gillian Greenberg, who had worked on the trials since 1979 on secondment from the Department of Health, took over management of the trial and the GPRF until her return to the Department in 1987, when Professor Tom Meade, the director of EMCU, assumed direct responsibility for the GPRF.

Over the years the GPRF developed into a cohesive network of between 250 and 300 practices with a strong sense of identity. Regular meetings ensured that the GPs and nurses got to know other GPRF members and fostered good relationships with the researchers at EMCU. One of the keys to the success of the GPRF was the involvement of nurses who were responsible for the day-to-day conduct of studies. Most nurses were practice nurses, though some were recruited specifically for trial work. The nurses were trained and supported by senior nurses, led in the early days by Greta Barnes, whose organisational skills contributed to the reputation the trials acquired for being run efficiently, and later by Wendy Browne. The regionally based senior nurses were also responsible for quality control. Another factor in the GPRF's success was efficient coordination by EMCU staff. The administration was headed in the early days by Sue Sinha who has since been joined by Claire Olohan-Bramley and Philip Roth.

In 1986, MRC decided that once the hypertension trials were completed the GPRF should continue as a national resource accessible to all researchers. It took some time for the research community to realise the potential of the Framework and in the late 1980s and early 1990s most of the research was initiated by the EMCU, Tom Meade's thrombosis prevention trial, in particular, enabling the GPRF to remain as a cohesive network. Notable exceptions were the series of studies undertaken by Professor Anthony Mann from the Institute of Psychiatry, whose involvement with the Framework continues today, and a study on diet and cholesterol initiated at the suggestion of the Framework GPs and conducted by Dr Paul Roderick while a public health trainee at the EMCU.

One of the possible reasons why the GPRF was then used by relatively few researchers was its perceived lack of representativeness. The preferred practice profile for the hypertension trials had been large with a stable patient population so that reasonable numbers of patients would be available for the duration of the trials and costs could be contained. To ensure that the GPRF could realise its potential a second recruitment drive was begun in 1992 for practices of types and in areas which were under-represented and also with the intention of expanding the GPRF overall to enable several large national trials and also regionally based research to be accommodated. A target of 850 practices in total was set, requiring the recruitment of around 600 new practices.

This second phase of development was coordinated by Dr Madge Vickers who now manages the GPRF. The starting point was lists of practices from the English family health service authorities (FHSAs) and from the Scottish, Welsh and Northern Ireland Offices. Some FHSAs were reluctant to provide lists but agreed to circulate information. The approach was similar to that used by Bill Miall:

- 8880 practices were sent a brief letter outlining plans
- 1908 practices responded requesting further information
- 913 practices were visited, mostly by a senior training nurse
- 656 new practices joined the GPRF.

Once again the enthusiasm of general practices was underestimated and the target was easily exceeded. This structured recruitment was and will continue to be supplemented by recommendations via personal contact with existing members and researchers involved in the Framework.

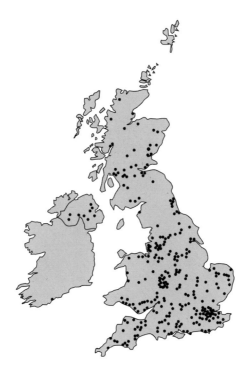

Figure 3.1 Location of GPRF practices

THE GPRF TODAY

Over 900 general practices throughout the UK, just over 8% of the total, are now associated with the Framework and together they access almost 11% of the UK population. Their location is shown in Figure 3.1. Table 3.1 gives the proportion of the practices and the population accessible, by region. Recruitment was successful across the whole spectrum of practice types including those previously under-represented:

• smaller practices
• practices in deprived areas and inner cities
• practices in Scotland, Wales, Northern Ireland and the North of England.

The composition of the Framework will never mirror that of UK general practices overall, but there are now sufficient practices of all types and in all areas to provide representative practice samples where necessary and this has been done in two major studies so far. Of equal importance, the characteristics of GPRF patients appear to follow UK population norms.

The second wave of practices share the enthusiasm of the earlier recruits for involvement in research, answering what they see as important clinical questions.

Table 3.1 The number and proportion of general practices that are GPRF members and the population accessed by region

Region (RHA or country)	Number of GPRF practices (% of region)	Population accessible (k) (% of region)
East Anglian & Oxford	104 (13.4)	882 (16.2)
South West	134 (13.3)	1014 (15.2)
South Thames	113 (8.8)	871 (12.2)
North Thames	84 (5.3)	560 (7.4)
West Midlands	71 (6.8)	529 (9.7)
Trent	76 (8.6)	501 (9.7)
North East and Yorkshire	78 (7.2)	616 (9.6)
North West	82 (6.1)	509 (7.5)
England	742 (8.2)	5483 (10.8)
Northern Ireland	36 (6.8)	255 (8.5)
Scotland	91 (8.4)	559 (10.4)
Wales	33 (9.3)	164 (9.4)
UK	902 (8.2)	6461 (10.6)

Both GPs and nurses enjoy the opportunity to interact with colleagues from other practices and researchers from many disciplines. The experience of research and training in research methodology is also considered valuable.

Terms of reference

- To serve as a national resource to undertake studies that require a coordinated framework of general practices.
- To facilitate research training of clinicians (including professions allied to medicine (PAMs)) and non-clinicians in health services research in primary care, with a view to improving their research and analytical skills.
- To provide a means for disseminating the results of research conducted within the GPRF and to promote implementation where appropriate.
- Through the coordinating centre:
  - to be responsive to MRC strategies in primary care research and, where appropriate, to broader national needs for research priorities in primary care including the developing NHS R&D programme for research in primary care
  - to serve as a means of identifying problems in primary care which may be accessible to research.

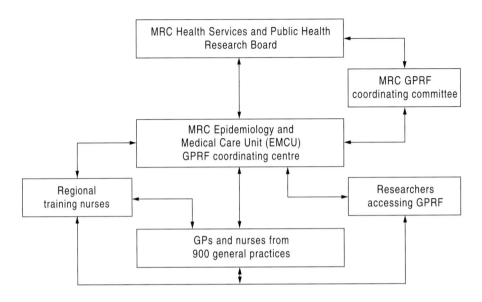

Figure 3.2   Interaction between the groups involved in GPRF research

Organisation of the Framework

The interaction between the groups involved in GPRF research is shown schematically in Figure 3.2. The key features are as follows.

General practices

- choose to participate only in studies of interest to practice
- provide invaluable feedback particularly during pilot studies
- influence research and other GPRF activities
- one GP per practice designated as contact doctor
- GP workload kept to minimum
- research (practice) nurse responsible for day-to-day management of studies
- nurses employed by practices
- nurse time at G grade and GP time for patient contact at NHS sessional rates reimbursed from MRC practice account with float of £2000
- monthly claims submitted to coordinating centre.

Regional training nurses

- senior nurses with experience of research (often in GPRF)
- first point of contact for practice nurses

- mostly based in and employed by GPRF practices
- often involved in pilot studies
- involved in initial group training sessions
- provide back up training at individual practices
- responsible for quality control in GPRF practices
- report to senior nurse manager (Ms Jeannett Martin) at EMCU.

Researchers

- from EMCU, universities, hospitals, research institutes, general practices and public bodies (e.g. Department of Health)
- peer-reviewed studies
- responsible for scientific direction, management, analysis and publication
- external researchers collaborate to varying degrees with EMCU staff.

Coordinating centre at EMCU

- responsible to MRC for infrastructure and management of GPRF
- responsible for financial monitoring and processing of claims for all studies
- select from interested practices to meet study requirements (e.g. geography, size, deprivation indices)
- responsible for work of training nurses
- holds and updates database of practice characteristics and research interests
- organises annual conference, regional meetings and specific study meetings
- prepares and distributes twice annual newsletter
- advises non-EMCU researchers, if appropriate, on protocol development, practical issues, study costings
- in collaborative studies may contribute statistical, study management, health economic and data processing input plus purchase and distribution of supplies
- in all studies, senior EMCU-based nurses provide backup for training and practice nurses
- scientific staff conduct much of their own research through the GPRF
- provides training opportunities for researchers (e.g. public health trainees, young scientists, GPs and nurses interested in epidemiology or health services research).

MRC GPRF coordinating committee

- independent MRC Committee
- monitors and oversees the work of the GPRF.

MRC Health Services and Public Health Research Board

- reviews activities of GPRF every five years
- provides staff and expenses for infrastructure
- receives an annual report from the GPRF coordinating committee.

Research in the GPRF

The GPRF has a deserved reputation for high-quality research founded on the successful conduct of the large, long-term clinical trials undertaken by Bill Miall, Gillian Greenberg, Tom Meade and their colleagues in the practices and at EMCU. Today the same principles are applied to a range of study types and sizes, namely:

- multidisciplinary collaboration
- thorough feasibility work
- close involvement of and consultation with GPs and nurses
- well established organisational procedures
- quality control by regionally based senior nurses
- regular feedback to practices.

In 1997 there were 23 GPRF studies:

- 14 trials involving between 5 and 450 practices
- 3 observational studies
- 2 studies of the genetic basis of disease
- 3 of patient management
- 1 of patients' access to services.

Six studies are EMCU initiatives, two are collaborative studies initiated externally but wholly managed by the Unit and 15 are externally initiated and managed. Topics covered include:

- cardiovascular disease
- hormone replacement therapy
- asthma
- back pain
- depression and anxiety
- management of elderly people
- infectious intestinal disease
- vitamin supplementation
- care of Alzheimer's patients
- implementation of research findings.

The variety of topics and the range of study types are increasing as the facilities offered by the GPRF are becoming more widely known and we are always keen to take on new studies. New practices are also welcome, whether they are new to research or would like to expand their current research activities. The following section describes the experience of two of the first GPRF members. Not all nurses and GPs will wish to follow the same path but the opportunities are there.

Box 3.1   MRC General Practice Research Framework
- Set up 1973, expanded 1992
- 900 practices
- Multicentre epidemiology and health services research
- Coordinated by MRC Epidemiology and Medical Care Unit
- Accessible to all researchers
- Projects peer-reviewed and funded
- Day-to-day management by practice nurses
- Established administrative procedures
- Training and quality control by senior regional nurses

A view from the grassroots

Lesley Hand and Christopher Hand

How we became interested

When we joined the MRC GPRF in 1978, LH was the mother of two small boys with another child on the way, and CH had been in practice at the Beeches in Bungay, for just two years. Neither of us had done any research before, and both our training backgrounds were predominantly in hospital medicine. It was also at a time when GPs could not get reimbursement for employing their wives in the practice.

The advertisement for MRC research practices appeared in the *BMJ* and it was our senior partner, Wyndham Jordan, who suggested that we should apply. He had an encyclopaedic knowledge of his patients and a keen eye for the unusual clinical presentation. He described the first case in the British literature of pulmonary embolism on the oral contraceptive pill, in a simple letter to the *Lancet*.[1] His interest in, and enthusiasm for, research acted as a catalyst for our application.

The practice

The Beeches was a four-man practice with 10 000 patients in a small market town on the borders of Norfolk and Suffolk. We employed two nurses and had a health visitor, two district nurses and two midwives attached to the practice. We had an age–sex register and a well-organised system for immunisation, but no screening programmes. We ran a mixture of appointment and open surgeries, but special clinics for chronic diseases were not in existence. Our premises had just been updated and we had some free space on the third floor.

Getting started

Before being accepted into the Framework, we were visited by Bill Miall and invited to Stratford-upon-Avon to be vetted by Greta Barnes. We then went to visit Anthony White in Newmarket, whose practice was one of the first to join the Framework (clinic 32). We became clinic 66.

What we've done

Our first trial

We were involved in the first trial that the GPRF undertook: the mild hypertension trial. This involved screening the blood pressures of all the men and women in the practice from the age of 35 to 64. We sent for the patients in alphabetical order, with the unexpected effect of family reunions occurring in the waiting room! The response rate was also unexpected: 92%. We were amazed at the patients' interest in the study, and their commitment to taking part in clinical trials remains a key factor to this day. The research process also set the scene for the practice screening programmes and the nurse-run clinics that preceded the new contract by over a decade.

Other trials

The elderly hypertension trial came next and it was a real treat meeting healthy over-65-year-olds. It is all too easy to forget that most people are well when bogged down by everyday practice. The other studies we have been involved with are:

- thrombosis prevention trial
- lifestyle and health intervention study
- feasibility study for the hormone replacement therapy trial
- the effect of stress in the workplace on health
- pilot study of testing for microalbuminuria in diabetics in general practice
- nurse support in the management of depression study
- antidepressants and self-help in the treatment of mild depression

- assessment of long-term efficacy of early introduction of inhaled steroids in asthma pilot
- bezafibrate in the treatment of lower arterial disease.

The list illustrates the broad range of interest that involvement in the Framework brings. There were several other trials that we would have liked to have done, but we simply did not have the time.

The annual conference

One big advantage of being in the Framework is the opportunity to meet like-minded people from all over the UK at the annual conference. When we first joined, the conference had moved to Churchill College, Cambridge, where the combination of the surroundings and the excitement of hearing authorities speak was very stimulating. Perhaps the most exciting thing of all was when results were presented; we could see the fruits of our work.

The Framework has become so successful that it has had to move from Cambridge to other venues to accommodate the extra members. This has resulted in some loss of intimacy, but the introduction of workshops at the conference and the development of regional meetings have partly addressed this issue.

The effects on personal development

The nurse's view

Most of my post-registration experience had been on medical wards. I had never worked as a practice nurse nor done any research. The post of MRC trial nurse seemed to offer a challenging opportunity to combine these two roles.

The diversity of the research projects undertaken by MRC has naturally resulted in the acquisition of valuable knowledge and skills. The two hypertension trials and the thrombosis prevention trial focused on the need to identify patients at risk from coronary heart disease and stroke. Trying to encourage behavioural change in the overweight, hypertensive smoker who enjoyed the euphemistic 'odd pint' was not easy. However, one huge benefit of undertaking this type of research in a primary care setting is the rapport that builds up over time between the nurse and the participants. They see me several times a year and even if they are not particularly motivated to change their lifestyle at the first interview, they sometimes do so during follow up.

Later studies included a prospective study of the use of hormone replacement therapy and its effect on breast cancer, osteoporosis and cardiovascular events. Again there was ample scope for using the enhanced knowledge about these conditions in daily practice.

Becoming a practice nurse

In 1990, having worked as an MRC nurse for 12 years, I joined the practice to help them with the changes enforced by the new contract. Practice nursing was then a speciality for which much of the training was experiential. I have to say that without the background of my MRC work, I would have been completely stuck.

Developing psychological skills

As the Framework continued to expand, other organisations saw its potential for clinical research. The Institute of Psychiatry conducted a nurse support study in the treatment of mild depression, and Bungay was one of 20 clinics that took part. The training I received in the recognition and treatment of depression, impinged on all aspects of my practice workload. As a student nurse there was very limited availability for placements in the psychiatric unit, which resulted in a lack of training in this field.

Becoming a regional nurse trainer

After six years working in Bungay, I became a regional nurse trainer covering the East Anglian and North Thames regions. This provided me with the chance to see at first hand how the studies are carried out in individual practices. Whereas sometimes there may be a lack of space or time, there is never a lack of enthusiasm. Part of my job means that I am often the first personal contact for the Framework when I arrive to explain the recruitment process. It is not unusual to meet what seems to be the entire primary care team, reflecting the level of interest in primary care research.

Many of the MRC nurses are practice nurses. Taking on additional work, especially after the demise of health promotion clinics, has been welcomed. The flexibility of working within the Framework ensures that the extra hours fit easily with practice and personal commitments, and the two roles constantly intertwine. Meeting so many practice nurses and becoming aware of their professional development encouraged me to start as a nurse mentor for Suffolk Health. Nursing research and audit are developing rapidly: more nurses are now performing their own projects as part of degree courses, and my increased knowledge of research methods gleaned from the MRC trials has been invaluable.

Doing my own research

The deep pool of expertise on tap at the Wolfson Institute and the excitement engendered by study results, have made me consider undertaking some qualitative research looking into practice nurse training needs. In addition to my senior nurse manager, Jeannett Martin, who has published widely in the nursing press, there are statisticians, epidemiologists, psychologists and research assistants available to help with the development of projects. Having contact with people in other health disciplines has been one of the most stimulating aspects of the job.

The doctor's view

Having collaborated in research, I wanted to realise an ambition to do some research myself. The stimulus came in 1990 with the imposition of the new contract. My response was to go and do an MSc in general practice at Guy's Hospital. This course radically changed my thinking about medicine, let alone general practice, and undertaking a research project was by far the most challenging thing I had done since becoming a GP.

After completing the MSc, I became an associate adviser for postgraduate general practice. This position gave me the opportunity to develop educational links between the University of East Anglia and general practice. A year later, a multidisciplinary MSc in Health Sciences was launched, and there are now over 180 students from a wide variety of health professions taking part. Many of them are doing research projects of their own.

During this time, I undertook a qualitative study into the monitoring of hospital training by Royal Colleges,[2] and continued the work that I had started on my MSc.[3] Working with a clinical psychologist enabled me to obtain my first research grant from the regional health services research subcommittee. The proposal was to develop a measure for assessing patients' adherence to inhaler treatment for asthma.

It was at this point that Professor Weiman from Guy's Hospital approached me to join a multidisciplinary team to study patients' attitudes to asthma and its treatment. Such a study needed a representative sample of patients and so we decided to involve the GPRF. My research cycle had come full circle and I found myself helping to plan a research project for the Framework that I had joined nearly 20 years before.

The effects on the practice

The effects on the practice have been less tangible as the responsibility for the work falls mainly on one nurse and one doctor. It has, however, demonstrated that research that is properly resourced can go on in our practice without disrupting the day-to-day clinical work. This experience will be important when the practice applies to become one of the new regional research practices and joins the developing primary care research networks in Norfolk and Suffolk.

The effects on the patients

The MRC studies have involved a significant proportion of our patients and have generated a considerable amount of goodwill. Those patients who actually take part in the studies appreciate the extra care they receive. They recognise, however, that although they may not benefit individually, they may help others by their participation. This generous attitude is a pleasant contrast to the all too common view of patients as demanding individuals with ever increasing expectations.

The relationship between the GPRF and the developing primary care research networks

Although the GPRF has been in existence for 25 years, smaller primary care networks are now becoming more prominent. The development of primary care research is being actively encouraged, and it is going to be very important for the Framework to communicate with the newer networks. There are going to be opportunities to involve even more primary care professionals in research and this will need to be carefully coordinated.

There needs to be a balance between small-scale research done for personal interest and professional development, and grand multicentre research that answers questions of national importance. We think that the key to success lies with involving individuals in both types of research.

REFERENCES

1. Jordan WMJ (1961) Pulmonary embolism. *Lancet.* **2**: 1146–7.

2. Hand CH (1994) Joint hospital visiting: problems and solutions. *Postgraduate Education for General Practice.* **5**: 247–53.

3. Hand CH and Bradley C (1996) Health beliefs of adults with asthma: toward an understanding of the difference between symptomatic and preventive use of inhaler treatment. *Journal of Asthma.* **33**: 331–8.

4

Research practices

Jim Cox and Andrew Farmer

Research practices are NHS general medical practices with at least one partner who is an experienced primary care researcher. Research practices may be funded to provide protected research time for the lead general practitioner, a research assistant, secretarial support or other running costs.[1] The purpose of this chapter is to describe the opportunities that exist for those who wish to move towards becoming a research practice and to look at the practical issues involved.

Research practices are a logical component of a primary care-led NHS which is intended to lead to a move of care, education and resources into the community. To carry out primary care research relevant to clinical practice, clinicians and other health care professionals are needed with a background in research, appropriate training and the opportunity to continue in practice.[2]

Most patient contact takes place in primary care and although research in primary care can be carried out by university-based researchers, active involvement of those working in practice should result in more valid and relevant questions being asked and answered.[3] Like GP training practices, research practices are autonomous but accountable to the body that funds them. Although they are independent of university departments of general practice, strong links between research practices and academic institutions facilitate access to the range of multidisciplinary skills, such as statistics, health service research, psychology and sociology, which are essential for high quality research. Collaborative working with other disciplines is more likely to produce and develop successful ideas and projects than is the occasional consultative use of their services.

Becoming a research practice offers a forward-looking primary healthcare team the opportunity to establish a training structure within the practice that will be of continuing benefit to partners, nurses, ancillary staff, registrars and students. The structure also offers the opportunity for those interested to undertake higher research degrees while based in the practice. Shared interest in research encourages success in what is often a difficult and isolated experience. Team members wishing to pursue research can maintain their interest. Funding enables pre-protocol research and the employment of research assistants and secretaries.

Active involvement in research is also a stimulus to critical examination of day-to-day clinical care, encouraging a way of thinking that is receptive to new ideas, while maintaining an ability to critically evaluate their application.

Becoming a research practice is a challenge. As an isolated interest of a single team member it offers the group no advantages. The disruptive effect of a solitary individual trying to engage in research within a partnership inevitably leads to tensions. However, when a whole healthcare team has a shared vision which includes an active research commitment, then undertaking research alongside providing patient care can improve job satisfaction, teamwork and clinical care. It should also provide new knowledge for the wider benefit of general practice and primary healthcare.

WHO APPOINTS RESEARCH PRACTICES?

The first research practices were appointed by the Royal College of General Practitioners (RCGP) in October 1994. They were paid £4500 per year for three years, not as a research grant but as 'pump priming' money to stimulate research within the practice. Since then the College has appointed other practices around the UK, the main aim being to encourage other organisations, particularly NHS regional research and development directorates, to follow suit.

Funding is intended to enable the practices to develop a research infrastructure, for example by employing additional staff, 'buying' time for a doctor to devote to research and purchasing computer hardware and software. The current rate (in 1997) is about £15 000 per year, which does not go very far. Research practices, like other researchers, must attract money for their projects.

Many practices with a research capacity have bid for funding under the NHS levy for research and development arrangements. The model of a research practice should be attractive to those offering funding because it provides an established structure within which to manage a budget for research work carried out as part of an NHS commitment. As arrangements for this funding become more secure, the role of the RCGP and NHS regions may shift to one of accrediting the standards of research practices rather than in providing direct funding.

Criteria for appointment to one of the formal schemes vary but may include some of the following:

- possession by the lead partner of a higher research degree by thesis, such as an MSc, MD or PhD, or a firm intention to obtain one
- previous research grant awards
- publications in peer-reviewed journals
- adequate computer equipment, expertise and support
- commitment to research by the practice as a whole

- applicants should be in active general practice
- preparedness to encourage and support research locally.

Research practices should be active general practices with a corporate commitment to research. Although links with universities are desirable, research practices should not be part of university departments or led by senior academics.

LINKING WITH OTHER ORGANISATIONS

Research is no longer a solitary occupation. Primary healthcare research has developed into a discipline with its own body of literature and methods. It has encouraged examination of problems from multiprofessional perspectives, including nursing, and adopted research methods from other disciplines, e.g. the qualitative methods used by sociologists and psychologists. A research practice can benefit by adopting these principles. The precise needs of an individual practice will vary. A practice may have members with sufficient time available and a sufficiently varied set of backgrounds and research experience to undertake substantial amounts of research activity without the need for outside links. However, most practices will need to have strong links with universities. Participation in medical student teaching, previous involvement in research and registration for a research degree or course may all help.

Advice is available from a number of sources. Most NHS regions now have research networks in place to link researchers and provide advice to those interested in developing their skills and ideas. Contact with the RCGP through their research network is another means of maintaining links with others in a similar position.

MANAGING THE RESEARCH PRACTICE

Research practices normally have a 'lead partner' for research – the person whose name headed their application to become a research practice and who is accountable for its research activities.

Some practices have a small steering group to guide and advise on strategy, projects and funding. Members may be experienced academic researchers, perhaps from a local university. Meeting say twice a year, a steering group can help to determine policy as well as strengthening links between the practice and academic departments. Steering group members may also be willing to read and criticise draft documents such as project protocols, bids for funding and papers to be submitted for publication.

It is helpful to have a management group within the practice, meeting perhaps weekly to oversee and take responsibility for day-to-day research activities. The group should be small but include the lead partner, another member of the practice team (e.g. nurse), a research assistant and the person responsible for managing the budget.

Managing the budget

It is important that research income and expenditure can be clearly identified. Whether this is done within the practice accounts or as a separate account is up to the individual practice, but sound financial management is essential. The practice needs to know to what extent it is subsidising research (and it usually is). Funding agencies (including both the organisation which appointed the research practice and grant providers) are also entitled to know how their money is being spent. The practice manager, or whoever is responsible for managing the budget, should produce regular financial forecasts and a complete annual account.

Deciding on projects

It is sensible to have some idea of a focus for research before applying to become a research practice. The lead applicant is likely to have a prior track record of peer-reviewed research which he or she might wish to continue and develop. Faced with a number of possible projects, decisions need to be made on priorities. Start slowly and build on experience rather than trying to write large numbers of grant applications in different areas. With a developing track record, well presented ideas and patience, funding is likely to be found at some point.

The next problem is actually carrying out the project. Although responsibility for monitoring and managing a research project remains with the grant applicant, a researcher assistant who is working for a PhD or a post-doctoral research worker can undertake much of the work. Strong university links are again desirable to attract high quality personnel. However, to gain credibility for obtaining grants which involve employing others to carry out the day-to-day aspects of research, there is a need for both a track record in research and the availability of protected time in which to manage and supervise those conducting the research.

Other issues include the feasibility of projects within general practice. To achieve sufficient patient numbers, many worthwhile studies will involve collaboration with surrounding practices, or even those from further afield.

Projects involving large numbers of professional people, e.g. in professional consensus development, are unlikely to be successful. The numbers involved and the range of collaborating disciplines make this type of research more suited to full-time workers. There are no advantages in basing this type of research in a clinical setting.

Obtaining grants

With an established infrastructure for research, the next step is to obtain funding for individual studies. Funding for grants is available from a wide range of sources. Each regional NHS Executive Research and Development Division has a budget for researchers. The Clare Wand Fund of the British Medical Association, the Scientific Foundation Board of the RCGP and a number of other charities including the British Heart Foundation, the Stroke Association and the British Diabetic Association also have grant money available. Larger sums of funding for well designed studies are available from the National R&D Programme, provided that the project is within one of its defined areas of interest. The Wellcome Trust or the Medical Research Council may fund studies of disease mechanisms or basic science if applied for in collaboration with a university department.

The Northern and Yorkshire R&D office publishes a directory of potential research funding sources.

INTERDISCIPLINARY/TEAMWORK

Some of the most satisfying primary care research projects involve two or more professional disciplines. Primary healthcare is a multidisciplinary activity and this should be reflected in practice research activities. Joint learning of research methods and working together on individual projects can strengthen professional relationships within a practice, with benefit to all concerned, not least patients.

Ideas for new projects from all members of the practice team should be sought and encouraged. Training in research methods can be organised within the practice (perhaps based on constructive criticism of draft proposals), and sought through research networks and attendance at courses run by universities and other bodies.

The research practice management group should not only include interested doctors. The group has a leadership responsibility – to stimulate as many people as possible to learn about research through participation, not only by collecting data but also by working through their own ideas.

VISITORS

Because one of their functions is to 'fly the flag' for primary care research, research practices appointed by the RCGP are expected to make themselves available to receive visitors, such as College contacts or other interested parties, who wish to see research in action in an NHS general practice. Far from being a burden, it is an enjoyable and stimulating privilege to discuss the concept of research practices with its advantages, disadvantages, opportunities, pitfalls, ups and downs, etc., as well as individual projects with visitors. As well as local NHSE, academic and health authority visitors, British research practices have welcomed several research students and visiting academics from abroad, particularly the USA.

OUTCOMES (E.G. PUBLICATIONS, PRESENTATIONS, HIGHER DEGREES)

A research practice intent on garnering future funding must ensure that it achieves measurable outcomes. For example, an important outcome may be a practice team member obtaining a higher research degree. This will help to establish credibility with funding bodies and open the way to supervising other people working for such degrees. Presentations at conferences are also important since personal contacts with other researchers, academics and funding agencies help to create a good impression of the practice, its personnel and its work. Publications of papers, review articles and letters in peer-reviewed literature are also tangible measures of quality research activity.

Any primary care researcher willing to put their head above the parapet, however, is likely to be subjected to constant requests to offer consultative advice, undertake educational activities and to represent groups. Be selective!

CONCLUSIONS

Undertaking the development of a research practice is a rewarding but demanding task. As the direction of primary care research in the UK becomes clearer[4] the combined expertise of those already involved in practice-based research will provide further guidance. The best research practices will provide the highest standards of scientific rigour in their studies, with strong links with academic departments, other research practices and with their colleagues in service practice. Research practices will provide a scientific underpinning and model for day-to-day practice.

REFERENCES

1. Smith LFP (1997) Research practices: what, who and why? *British Journal of General Practice.* **47**: 83–6.

2. Gray DP (1995) Research general practices. *British Journal of General Practice.* **45**: 516–17.

3. Van Weel C (1995) General practice: a suitable place for clinical research. *European Journal of General Practice*. **1**: 6–7.

4. Carter YH (1997) Funding research in primary care: is Culyer the remedy? *British Journal of General Practice*. **47**: 543–4.

Personal view

David Seamark

HONITON GROUP PRACTICE: AN NHS RESEARCH PRACTICE

Practice profile

The Honiton Group Practice comprises two partnerships working from a purpose-built premises in a semi-rural market town in East Devon. There are 11 partners ($8\frac{1}{2}$ full-time equivalents) with a practice population approaching 15 000. The group practice is on the same site as the community hospital which contains general practitioner beds, a minor injuries unit, maternity unit, elderly confused unit and outpatient and diagnostic facilities. The hospital is covered by the partners and is also the treatment centre of the East Devon Out-of-Hours Co-operative.

The practice has invested heavily in information technology and effectively became 'paperless' in 1990. Personal computers with Windows running the Exeter System were introduced in 1994. One partner has been involved in developing the software and the practice has frequently piloted new software, the latest being Path Links (automatic download of pathology laboratory results from Exeter).

My personal background was a scientific training in Biochemistry followed by a PhD in Chemical Pathology, before reading Medicine. After completing vocational training I recommenced my research career in the field of palliative medicine. Initially a research fellow in the Institute of General Practice of the University of Exeter, I became a part-time lecturer in 1995; I had been careful since starting as a full-time partner to preserve a four day week commitment with two sessions of protected research time.

Research practice status

It was in 1994 that the first wave research practices funded by the RCGP were appointed. Until then my own research career had been centred on the academic department in Exeter, but another partner in Honiton (my wife Clare Seamark!) had started a research project using the Honiton database. Her work looked at contraceptive uptake by teenagers and teenage pregnancies and led to her registering for an MPhil. The concept of basing research firmly in the practice became more appealing as we realised that so much of the computerised clinical data was under-used and could lend itself to research. The second wave of RCGP research practices were advertised and after discussion with all the partners it was felt that it was the right time to apply. Our strengths were a large stable practice population, being monopoly suppliers of healthcare (through the practice and the hospital), our high degree of computerisation and commitment to audit and having two partners already involved in research. Weaknesses centred around our numerous commitments within practice and hospital, our distance from the resources such as medical libraries and academic departments, and little idea how to organise a research programme within a working surgery.

We were appointed in October 1995 as an RCGP research practice with a contract running for two years. This length of commitment was less than ideal, but fortunately the South & West NHS Region took up the concept of research practices and accepted Honiton on to their scheme in 1997. This in turn led to the 'invitation' to bid for Culyer NHS Research Funding. I endured the tortuous process of filling in the application form and Honiton was fortunate in being awarded Culyer Funding for four years running from April 1998.

DIFFICULTIES AND CHALLENGES ENCOUNTERED WITH RESEARCH PRACTICE STATUS

Which model to introduce?

There appear to be two models emerging. On is that of the individual researcher who gratefully accepts protected research time, perhaps employs a research assistant, but essentially works in isolation on projects of particular personal interest. This model has certain advantages of being focused, simple to organise administratively, but disadvantages of possible professional isolation and perhaps some opposition from other members of the primary health care team (PHCT) who would like to be involved. The other model, which we have adopted at Honiton, is for the lead research GP to act as facilitator and manager of the overall research effort of the practice. This has advantages of enabling more members of the PHCT to become involved, builds wider contacts with other agencies and perhaps engenders greater ownership of the research culture in the practice. The disadvantages are that it can be hard to be as focused in research topics, supervision is time consuming, administration is more complex and the skills of an experienced researcher under-employed through lack of time. I will enlarge on some of these problems.

Administration

To a partner not normally involved in the finer details of practice management, administering a research budget can be quite a headache. I have found keeping track of expenditure from a number of different research budgets difficult and due to lack of training, unnecessarily time consuming. If the practice research effort is large and increasing it requires training and perhaps sub-contracting the financial responsibilities to another person, or perhaps to an academic unit, used to handling such affairs. For our practice manager the research accounts have been conceptually difficult to understand (what exactly is infrastructure support, non-externally funded research, etc.?) and a substantial additional workload.

Employing staff for research has proved challenging. Does one employ staff already working in the practice and hence familiar with the other staff and computerised databases, or advertise formally? What is the job description of someone working in a new field with fluctuating workload? Who is to employ the researcher – all the partners or just the lead researcher? We have had to tackle the problem of employing new staff at a time when the demise of fundholding may well lead to redundancies in the practice. Employing staff normally employed in the surgery to do research work extra to their routine commitments (such as practice nursing and phlebotomy) but within normal working hours requires careful drawing up of job descriptions and calculation of remuneration.

Paperwork for me has escalated rapidly. With funding comes responsibilities that as an employee of a university, I have not generally been faced with. Grant giving bodies use a different language and I would quote the opaque guidance of the Culyer application as an example. I have had to learn how to interpret guidance, requests for information, invitations to bid for funds, etc. with a view to a hidden agenda.

Staff development

With more staff in the surgery being involved in research our deficiencies in training becomes more apparent. Having undergone a formal research training it is not a problem I have faced before. Two partners have taken the route of registering for an MPhil and receiving formal supervision. For staff not at that level it has been more difficult and more *ad hoc*. How does one select one practice nurse over another for further funded training in research methodology and not alienate her colleagues? How able are research naive colleagues to discern their educational needs? This is an area in which I could use some help and guidance.

Fortunately, through academic units and regional research and development directorates such help is now available.

Protected time

Everyone complains of lack of time. The research practice funding provides the invaluable commodity of protected time. I have found the time increasingly used in administration and time for 'real' research being confined to my time off. This is inevitable in a practice that has taken to research with enthusiasm and is probably a price worth paying, at least in the initial phase of consolidating, i.e. publishing results and obtaining grants.

BENEFITS OF BEING A RESEARCH PRACTICE

Fun

It's fun, stimulating and a wonderful tonic for the jaded partner and PHCT members who feel their potential is unfulfilled. I have been gratified by the way many members of the practice have taken on the research ethos. Of the 11 partners seven are actively involved in research projects. One former receptionist, having taken an Access course and a degree in psychology, has returned to work as a research assistant for the practice. She is developing her career in research in what I consider a novel way and she brings a completely different perspective to the projects we have started.

Flexibility

The protected time has been beneficial for me personally, but the ability to provide time for staff to work ideas up into proposals has also been very helpful. The provision of a few locum sessions or paying a member of staff to visit another practice or institution greatly speeds up the process of project development.

Practice infrastructure

The on-cost element in the research budget is of benefit to the practice in improving the computerised database, covering the costs of extra postage, photocopying, telephone bills and room space. The subscriptions to various journals and the Internet connections have served to bring the evidence base of medicine more firmly into the practice.

Networking

Research practice status has greatly increased our profile and consequently attracts visitors and invitations to participate in other research. The collaboration with other agencies has been stimulating in that new skills and concepts are introduced and the robustness of projects enhanced.

Sense of purpose

Every general practice wishes to serve patients to the best of its ability. Research has enabled us to fulfil this in a different manner. We have found our patients very enthusiastic about participating in research and there is a sense of local pride that we are involved in improving healthcare.

CONCLUSIONS

Research practice status is well worth achieving, but it is important that the whole practice is in agreement with the decision and on the model the lead research GP chooses to work to. The amount of time and complexity of administering a research budget should not be underestimated. The managing of staff and their personal development requires expertise that may not initially be present in the practice.

5

Research training fellowships

Bonnie Sibbald

BACKGROUND

The development of primary healthcare has been handicapped by a long-standing dearth of high-quality research. The reasons for this are complex but certainly include a lack of research training among primary healthcare professionals. The need to provide better research training opportunities has long been recognised, but active interventions to change the situation did not gather momentum until the late 1980s. The Royal College of General Practitioners (RCGP) was the first to introduce research training fellowships specifically targeted at general practitioners in 1987. This was followed in the early 1990s by the government's introduction of a service increment for teaching and research (SIFTR) equivalent for general practice which was used by most university departments of general practice to fund research training posts for general practitioners. Such initiatives have been advanced further in the mid-1990s by the NHS regional directors of research and development who have introduced bursaries and research training fellowships specifically targeted at primary healthcare professionals. Such is the importance now attached to research in primary healthcare that training fellowships are available from a wide range of sources, including the Royal Colleges, the national research councils, regional R&D offices of the NHS Executive and a number of major charities.

GOALS, AIMS AND OBJECTIVES

The ultimate goal for the organisations which sponsor research training fellow-ships is to improve the quality and cost-effectiveness of healthcare by enhancing research activity. Organisations aim to achieve this by providing training in research for healthcare professionals, thereby creating a larger body of people to contribute effectively to research. The specific objectives of any particular fellow-ship naturally vary with the sponsoring organisation. Most, however, broadly concur with those of the RCGP, which are to enable the fellow to:

- acquire research skills
- pursue an original line of enquiry
- pursue a higher research degree, usually MD or PhD
- be linked to an academic unit where there will be appropriate supervision.

Implicit within these goals, aims and objectives is the expectation that health pro-fessionals will use the fellowship to launch themselves on a longer-term career in research, or as professional 'leaders' able effectively to commission research and encourage its uptake into clinical practice. Indeed, the success of fellowship schemes is often judged, not simply in terms of satisfactory completion of training, but in terms of whether fellows continue to pursue a career in research and foster the development of research skills and awareness in others.

Box 5.1   Fellowships

- Provide protected time in which to
  - acquire research skills
  - conduct a research project
- Are targeted at people who
  - are practising clinicians
  - have some research experience
  - want a career in research

ARRANGEMENTS

Fellowships provide health professionals with protected time in which to under-take a programme of research training linked to the development and completion of a specific research project. The fellow is attached to a reputable academic unit, usually within a university, where their training and research is supervised by an experienced senior researcher. The training programme is tailored to the specific needs of the fellow and typically may comprise short, formal courses, personal one-to-one tuition and participation in the wider academic life of the university.

The research project is intended to facilitate the practical development and application of research skills, as well as advance knowledge about health or healthcare practice within a given field.

The nature and level of financial support provided by fellowships varies tremendously among sponsoring organisations. All fellowships aim to secure protected time for research by providing income to offset time away from clinical practice. However, the level and duration of support may vary from partial salary reimbursement for 2–4 sessions per week over a period of 1–2 years, to full salary reimbursement for full time work over 3 years. Fellowships also vary in which, if any, of the following 'optional extras' they will fund:

- registration fees for higher degrees
- funds to attend relevant training courses and/or conferences
- travel and subsistence for attending courses and/or conferences
- the running costs of the research project itself
- payments to offset the costs of the academic unit which hosts the fellow.

SELECTION PROCEDURES

Fellowships are competitive awards and the procedure for selecting the winning candidate varies from organisation to organisation. Some only consider written applications, while others additionally interview short-listed candidates. All award panels, however, focus on three principal factors in making their judgement – the quality of the proposed training, the quality of the candidate and the quality of the proposed research project. Candidates must be strong in all three areas if they are to succeed.

In judging the quality of the candidate, awards panels look for:

- evidence of excellence in undergraduate and postgraduate professional training (e.g. awards, distinctions, prizes, etc.)
- evidence of prior research experience. Preference is given to candidates who have had some experience in all or most phases of research from design to completion, and who have disseminated their research through publication and lectures
- how well the candidate's career trajectory fits with the objectives of the fellowships. Does the candidate's previous training and experience show a clear line of progression towards a career in research? How will the fellowship help to advance the candidate's career goals?
- statements from the candidate's referees suggesting that the candidate has the ability and commitment successfully to undertake the fellowship.

In judging the quality of the proposed training programme, awards panels examine:

- the academic credentials of the host institution and supervisor. Does the supervisor and host department have a good research track record? Does the proposed research fit with the supervisor's interests? How experienced is the supervisor in supervising higher degrees? Can the supervisor set aside adequate time for supervision?

- the ability of the proposed training programme to meet the fellow's needs and the demands of the proposed project. Specifically does the programme provide training in the research skills and methodologies needed to complete the proposed research project? Is access to and funding for the proposed training problematic?

In judging the quality of the research proposal, panels ask whether:

- the topic addressed is relevant and important to primary healthcare (or the sponsor's selected topic for support)
- the project offers suitable opportunities for expanding and developing the candidate's research skills
- the research aims are clearly stated
- the plan of investigation is capable of fulfilling the stated aims
- the project is feasible within the proposed resources and timetable
- consideration has been given to how the necessary permissions (e.g. ethical committees) and funds needed to carry out the research will be obtained.

Box 5.2   Winning a fellowship

Awards panels are looking for a:
- good academic CV from a candidate
- relevant training programme
- well designed research proposal

FACTORS AFFECTING SUCCESS

The long experience of the RCGP in providing research training fellowships for GPs suggests that the following factors, although not essential, can influence the likelihood of success.

Fellow

Although the supervisor and academic host unit are there to guide fellows, many opportunities for learning will be wasted if the fellow waits passively to be led. Fellows need to become self-directed in their learning and proactive in seeking out support and resources.

Fellowships demand a lot of hard work which often extends beyond the officially protected time allotted to this activity. Prospective fellows need therefore to consider whether they, and their families, are prepared to lose some of their leisure time to research. A supportive and stable home life is invaluable. The disruption experienced by people undergoing house moves, job moves or other major life changes often seriously impedes progress with a fellowship.

Fellows need the support, not only of their families, but also their colleagues in the practice. It can be difficult for practices to cope with the extra workload or loss of income which may result from the fellow's absence. In this respect, larger group practices are often better able to redistribute their workload and cope more easily with the fellow's reduced clinical commitment. Colleagues may become resentful or jealous of the fellow's time away from clinical practice. It is therefore important to try to bring back to the practice some of the benefits of widening research experience. These may be technical skills to facilitate audit or support computing, or knowledge of clinical advances of relevance and importance to the practice team.

Supervisor

Good academic supervision is crucial to success. Before they agree to work together, prospective supervisors and fellows should first get to know each other well enough to know whether they have any major clashes in personality or preferred learning/teaching styles. Supervisors should not be overcommitted and so unable to spend regular time with the fellow. The directors or heads of academic units are often very busy and fellows may find that closer supervision can be provided by a less senior member of academic staff. Another factor to consider is whether the fellow's research interests fit with those of the supervisor. A fellow is likely to get more and better supervision when he or she is working in an area in which the supervisor is also research active.

The initial acid test for a good working relationship is how well the prospective supervisor and fellow work together in preparing the fellowship application. Is the supervisor able to spend time with the fellow in discussing the details of the proposed research? Does the supervisor appraise the fellow's research training needs and offer guidance on how to put together a training package to meet those needs?

Host unit

Ideally, fellows should look to locate themselves in an academic unit which has the reputation for excellence in research, particularly within the fellow's field of interest. It will be helpful to read the unit's annual report to gain a better impression of the nature and extent of the ongoing teaching and research activity. Ask the prospective supervisor about who else within the unit would be interested in the fellow's research and what staff might be willing and able to meet specific training needs. For example, is there a statistician who would be willing to offer advice on data handling and analysis?

Ask also about the physical resources which would be available. Host units should ensure that they have the adequate resources to accommodate the fellow (e.g. desk, phone, computing facilities, library facilities, etc.). However, the pressure on accommodation in many academic units can be so great that fellows may have to share desks, phones or computers. Fellows will be wise to clarify these arrangements before proceeding with an application.

Ideally fellows should be geographically close to their host academic unit. This makes it far easier to maximise the time spent in the academic unit and so benefit from its wider resources. A fellow who can only visit very occasionally will miss out on the opportunities to widen their personal support network, extend their knowledge by attending lectures and seminars, and make maximum use of the knowledge and skills of the academic unit as a whole.

Box 5.3   Factors facilitating completion

Fellow
- proactive personal orientation
- stable and supportive home life
- supportive clinical practice

Supervisor
- experienced researcher
- shares fellow's interests
- able and willing to devote time

Host unit
- geographically close
- good research track record
- good resources/accommodation

Finances

Careful consideration needs to be given to the level of available funding and whether this will be adequate to offset the costs to fellows and their practices. Look into how the arrangements for payment may affect superannuation, national insurance and practice entitlements to reimbursement. It can be very helpful to speak to past and current fellows about their financial arrangements.

Ideally the fellowship should offer some kind of financial reimbursement to the host unit so that the fellows are seen as a positive asset and not a potential drain on resources. Fellows who are supported by schemes which do not reimburse host academic units should not, however, despair. It is important to remember that the unit gains academic 'Brownie points' from grant income brought in by the fellow and through increased numbers of publications.

Fellows and supervisors need to plan ahead and secure: (i) the running costs of the research; (ii) fees for higher degree registration; and (iii) the costs of training courses, where these are not covered by the fellowship. Lack of forward planning can be a major obstacle to progress. The running costs of the research can often be obtained through grant applications to professional bodies (such as the Scientific Foundation of the RCGP), regional NHS R&D funding schemes or charities. Applications need to be submitted well in advance of the intended starting date for the research since it not uncommonly takes 4 months or longer to get a decision. Higher degree registration fees may be waived if the host academic unit makes the fellow an honorary member of staff. Otherwise explore the opportunities for obtaining an internal university bursary to cover these fees. There are generally no charges for attending courses within the university where the fellow is registered for a higher degree. The fees for courses held elsewhere may sometimes be obtainable from regional R&D bursary schemes.

Box 5.4   Finances
- Available funds to meet fellow's needs
- Available funds to meet practice's needs
- Plans to meet outstanding costs are laid well in advance

Making the most of a research fellowship

Helen Lester and Jonathan Graffy

The main reasons people undertake research fellowships are to learn skills in research, to get funding for time to undertake a study and to further their professional and personal development.

CHOOSING TRAINING

There are a number of ways in which you can be proactive in organising your own research training. To take full advantage of the opportunities offered by the fellowship, you need to decide what training you need at an early stage. Research fellows attached to a medical school department may be able to take advantage of the informal training and formal courses run by their own departments or the university staff development unit. A number of excellent research training courses are advertised in the journals, on Internet web sites and of course by word of mouth. If there's a specific skill you want to learn, ask the local expert in the field you're interested in about their training.

Higher degrees

You may like to consider whether you want to register for a more formal degree course as part of your research training.

- A number of medical schools run taught MSc courses, often part time over a 2-year period. They may seem expensive (approximately £1500 per year), but they cover a wide range of core research skills.
- Registering for an MD or PhD is a further option. PhDs are increasingly encouraged by departments of general practice since they are more closely supervised than MDs. Both involve a significant commitment of time and energy and may also focus your research training too narrowly if undertaken at the start of your research training.

Whichever route or combination of routes you take, you need to keep your individual training needs and career intentions in mind.

Box 5.5 Choosing training

- Be proactive
- Prioritise your own training needs
- Use local expertise – courses/advice
- Investigate courses further afield
- Consider registering for a further or a higher degree

SUPERVISION AND MENTORSHIP

Support can be given in many different ways. 'Junior/MD support groups', lunch-time meetings and journal clubs as well as informal discussions about learning needs can all be an important part of developing as a researcher. These, however, should be adjuncts to, not instead of, more formal supervision, as described earlier in this chapter.

Mentoring appears to mean different things to different people and is frequently confused with supervision. The roles of a supervisor and a mentor should be separate and neither will be fulfilled properly if you try and use the same person for both.

Box 5.6   The roles of a mentor

- Confidante
- Life guide
- Impartial career adviser

THE RESEARCH PROJECT (FIGURE 5.1)

The key to a successful research project is asking the right question, but it can take some time to clarify exactly what you want to find out. You need to be clear why a particular topic interests you and initially it may be better to consider a number of options. Medline and other computer databases are so accessible that it's worth checking at the outset if your ideas are original or not. Talk your ideas over with colleagues and see if they think the subject is important enough for you to devote your time to. At this stage, don't be scared to change tack or start all over again – it's better than wasting 2 years researching something which isn't original or can't be answered with the study you have designed.

Executing a qualitative study

Qualitative research, which is multimethod in focus, can provide a unique insight into a problem or topic. Qualitative methods are particularly appropriate:

- to research a topic that is poorly understood or previously unexplored
- to describe the form and nature of complex phenomena
- to generate ideas and hypotheses
- to gain the patient's view of the world
- to research a sensitive topic that would be inaccessible using quantitative methods.

However, quantitative and qualitative methodologies are not mutually exclusive and can often be used together to complement the exploration of a topic. Qualitative methods embrace a variety of different techniques, e.g. interviewing using semi-structured or depth interviews or group work, direct or indirect observation studies. The proportion of time spent on data analysis is far longer than in quantitative studies – there is a cyclical interaction between data collection and analysis, with analysis informing subsequent phases of the data collection.

Qualitative analysis involves individual splashes of inspiration and insight, but needs to be transparent to others to be rigorous. It can be performed manually,

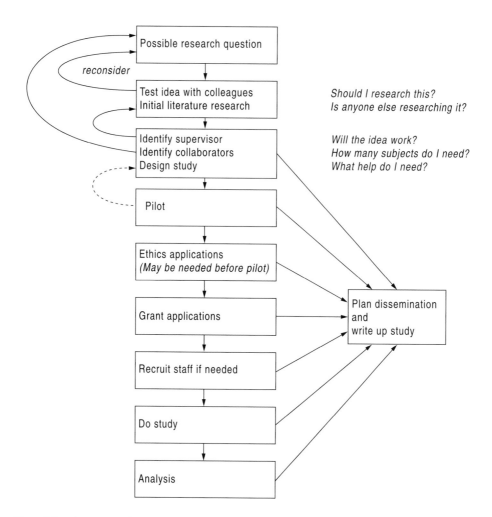

Figure 5.1 The research pathway

but increasingly there are computer packages that can assist with analysis. Once you've made the decision to use a qualitative approach, it's important to seek out appropriate training. I found out about training courses through my university behavioural science department and the Social Research Association. For more information about computer assisted analysis, I found CAQDAS network courses at the University of Surrey very useful.

Box 5.7   Checklist for qualitative studies

- Is the topic appropriate for a qualitative approach?
- Has appropriate training been sought?
- Is the methodology appropriate for the topic?
- Is the sampling clearly thought out and appropriate?
- Is there an iterative relationship between data analysis and collection?
- Is analysis rigorous and systematic, and supported by the data?
- Is the research trustworthy – is there evidence of member checking and searching for pieces of data that don't fit (disconfirming evidence)?
- Has the issue of generalisability been addressed?

Executing a quantitative study

While qualitative methods are useful in generating hypotheses and understanding a topic, researchers usually need to use a quantitative approach to test those ideas. The key difference for the person conducting the study is that whereas the qualitative researcher can learn about the topic and adapt his or her approach during the study, the quantitative researcher needs to iron out all the problems before recruiting any patients. The early stages of defining the research question, designing and testing questionnaires, getting statistical advice and piloting the study can take a year or two, but is time well spent.

The biggest problem doing the study is often keeping people interested and involved. It can take time to recruit large numbers of people and in that time staff may change or people may feel too busy to fill out yet another form. Keep encouraging those who are helping and look for new ways to reward their effort, whether with biscuits, champagne prize draws or a newsletter to tell them how the study is going. Never show your frustration, because you need their help more than they need your study.

Box 5.8   Checklist for Quantitative Studies

- Is the question worth asking?
- Are the aims of the study clearly stated?
- Is the study design capable of testing the hypotheses?
- How many subjects do you need? Can you recruit them?
- How will things be measured? Reliability and validity of instruments
- What could bias the results?
- Does the study pose ethical problems?
- How will you analyse results?

Data analysis is increasingly easy with computers, but cleaning, coding and entering data can take a lot of time and it is worth identifying someone to help with this. It is ironic that the computer may only take seconds to analyse the data you have taken so long to collect, but even at this stage, asking it the right questions is the key to getting the answers you want.

SURVIVING A RESEARCH FELLOWSHIP

The decision to take up a research fellowship inevitably affects your personal and practice life.

The practice

Reducing your hours can have a number of interesting effects on your practice. Our practice partners were very flexible and accepting of our request for a reduced clinical commitment. Practice staff and patients were understandably less forgiving. Retaining your clinical skills and maintaining a degree of continuity of care is possible, but taking up a research fellowship involves inevitable sacrifices in terms of breadth of clinical interests.

A little forward planning can help to ease some of these problems:

- Make sure some of your surgeries are unbooked.
- Take time to explain your new working pattern to practice staff.
- Work out coping mechanisms and replies for patients who consistently grumble about the lack of appointments.
- Make sure your postgraduate education allowance (PGEA) is from clinical courses and not solely research-related conferences.

Almost inevitably, the unpredictable nature of clinical work can encroach on research. It is therefore important to create a clear demarcation between your research and clinical time, which may be harder if your practice is also your research base.

Home life

Protected time for research is inevitably less structured and more immediately flexible than the daily routine of booked surgeries. However, grant application deadlines and conference presentations create their own time pressures, and the ability to work from home may mean you find your work encroaching more and more on personal or family time. Your partner's enthusiasm for your new job can be quickly tempered by dismay at the number of nights you then spend in the study!

If you're going to enjoy the fellowship and maintain a home life, you need to inform and involve your partner as much as possible:

- Ask and value their opinion before taking on new responsibilities.
- Be honest with yourself when offered new roles or tasks – are you saying yes simply because it sounds exciting, or because you're flattered to be asked? Is it a diversion from the real purpose of your research?

Personal sanity

If your practice and your partner are happy, then you can begin to enjoy the research fellowship. It can take a little time to grow used to the different atmosphere and pace of research.

- Never feel guilty that you've got time to read now.
- Collaborate with others. Learning as an apprentice in a research team and always having at least one project that's moving forward help to maintain motivation and morale.
- Involvement with a project you genuinely care about, where you want to discover the 'answer', is important in maintaining momentum.
- Research fellows are not immune to burn out – make time for yourself.

Box 5.9   Surviving the fellowship

- Plan ahead and prepare your practice for your changing role
- Maintain separate research and clinical days
- Consult your partner before taking on further roles and responsibilities
- Learn to say 'no'
- Make sure you're committed and enthusiastic about your research project
- Learn to collaborate with others
- Make time for yourself

USEFUL ADDRESSES

Social Research Association (SRA)
35 Buckingham Close
Ealing
London W5 1TS

Computer Assisted Qualitative Data Analysis Software (CAQDAS) URL:http://www.soc.surrey.ac.uk/caqdas/

Epidemiology for Clinicians Course
MRC Environmental Epidemiology Unit
University of Southampton
Southampton General Hospital SO16 6YD

6

Collaborative research in the Weekly Returns Service

Douglas Fleming

A research unit concerned with morbidity recording was visualised with the establishment of the College of General Practitioners.[1] The major step forward came in 1959 when the Nuffield Hospitals Trust provided financial support for the establishment of a College Records and Research Unit. The Unit was established to design and test methods of data collection within practices that would facilitate the use of data from general practice for epidemiological purposes. A particular concern at that time was the quality of the environment, and many of the members of the College active in establishing the Unit were also in an environmental study group known as 'Airs, Waters and Places'.

The research principle at the heart of these developments was that of reproducibility. For credibility, research findings must be reproducible and that means the methods must be well documented, capable of use in differing situations and at different times. Primary interest therefore lay in the need for standardised systems of data collection in practices. The coin of reproducibility has a reverse face – comparability – and standardised methods of data collection opened up opportunities for practices to compare with each other.

DESCRIBING THE CONSULTATION

Prior to the official establishment of the College Records Unit, officers of the College had been involved in the design and prosecution of the first general practice-based morbidity study.[2] In this study, doctors summarised the content of the consultation using diagnostic or, if not practicable, symptomatic terms compatible with the International Classification of Disease (ICD 7th edition). They also kept details of the occupation of the heads of households. This record card was stored in the medical record envelope and at the end of the study, removed for analysis. Though considerable information was made available about the health problems of patients consulting general practitioners, there was only limited opportunity for individual doctors or practices to analyse their own practice material. Nevertheless, there have been distinguished contributions to GP research using these methods. Among them, many of John Fry's contributions were based on the analysis of the summary card.

DIAGNOSTIC INDEX

The diagnostic index was introduced into general practice by Tev Eimerl[3] and gave a major boost to information gathering in primary care. The principle of consultation summary by diagnosis compatible with the ICD was maintained, but the added dimension of episode type was introduced. The episode is the primary basis for collecting data within the diagnostic index and it is essential for recorders to understand what constitutes a new episode of illness. The word implies a start and end point and that is not difficult to appreciate in the context of a hospital episode and has led to the development of hospital episode statistics. It is also not difficult to visualise in terms of services provided during a finite illness period, as for example might be associated with acute tonsillitis or even an inguinal hernia. However, there are difficulties when illnesses with a recurring character are considered: for example, peptic ulcer or depression. Doctors may disagree as to whether a person had overcome one episode of illness before describing the next as a new episode; rules defining the onset of episodes are therefore important. Asthma provides one of the most difficult examples. To investigate the impact of environmental factors on asthma, it is necessary to know when new episodes occur. In the Weekly Returns Service of the Royal College of General Practitioners (RCGP)[4] which is particularly concerned with the timing of new episodes of illness, a consultation in which a patient presents with an exacerbation of his asthma (as opposed to presenting solely for review or further medication) is described as a new episode. Similar, pragmatic rules are applied to other conditions.

When using the diagnostic index, home visits were distinguished from consultations on surgery premises, consultations prompting referral to a specialist were identified and amendments to diagnosis were clearly indicated. Referral and home visit data are particularly important in studies of health economics. Analysis of material stored in diagnostic indexes provides three levels of epidemiological study detail:

1 *Persons consulting* – persons consulting in a period is a measure of disease prevalence over that period (usually 12 months). It is a more important measure of illness in a community than cumulative prevalence, in which all persons who have ever had the illness are counted. The difference is strikingly contrasted when considering the prevalence of asthma. There is a very considerable difference

between the numbers of people who have ever experienced an attack of asthma (cumulative prevalence) and those experiencing asthma in a particular 12-month period (annual prevalence). The burden of asthma in the community is more closely reflected by the annual period prevalence than by the cumulative prevalence.

2 *Episode* – the number of episodes is the most useful statistic for measuring the overall burden of illness and for estimating resource provision. Additionally, as has been mentioned above, the episode can be allocated to a time for the purpose of studying seasonality and environmental factors, such as pollution and weather conditions.

3 *Consultation* – consultation statistics tell something of the interface between the community and the delivery of healthcare. There are large differences between consultation rates in different countries, partly relating to methods of remuneration and partly to the density of GPs. Sociodemographic factors influence consultation rates; the individual practice or practitioner and his style of interviewing patients is the key determinant.

COMPUTERISED INFORMATION SYSTEMS

During the last 15 years the diagnostic index has been eclipsed by computer-based information systems. Although these were introduced with little structure as to how diagnostic information would be stored, they have increasingly adopted the fundamental principles enshrined in the diagnostic index. The allocation of a consultation or episode type is necessary for analysing data. Consistency of recording is essential and experience from the general practice-based national morbidity studies and the Weekly Returns Service has shown that the discipline of recording from every consultation enhances the quality of recording. Computerised information systems in the UK store data in the form of Read codes,[5] which can be mapped to classification systems such as the International Classification of Disease. The beauty of Read codes lies in the considerable detail with which diagnostic information can be described. This is a particular advance in the field of medical information storage because the code can be used to identify the disease sufficiently precisely for medical management, yet remain in a form in which automated coding is possible.

THE IMPORTANCE OF A DEFINED POPULATION

The procedures for registration with a particular doctor have given GPs in the UK an advantage for conducting epidemiological surveys as compared with colleagues in other countries. With the development of group practices this advantage has been eroded slightly, but nevertheless a defined population is cared for by a defined group of doctors. To interpret information concerned with counts of persons, a denominator is needed to derive rates. The rules for governing the inclusion of patients in the denominator must be matched by those in the numerator. Thus it is usual in analysis of general practice-based data to count only those persons who are formally registered in the practice.

Historically, the first practice counts were based on age–sex register cards.[6] These defined the point of entry into the practice (registration) and the point of departure. They were maintained in the practices, who observed simple clerical routines to maintain accuracy. These have been completely replaced by computerised registers. It is now common for practices and health authorities to be working with agreed practice populations.

Age–sex denominators can be determined on any particular day. For example, for the analysis of data collected in the Weekly Returns Service, the population denominator is defined at the mid-point of the recording period. This method is acceptable for a study within a short defined period, but not acceptable for a study over a 12-month period. Many people are only registered in a practice for part of the year and it is necessary to take this into account when defining both numerator and denominator in epidemiological surveys. The analysis of the practice-based morbidity surveys has involved counting the population denominators each day and deriving an average for the year.[7]

Although the age and sex distribution of the population will always be the primary denominator for reporting general practice-based morbidity rates, there are some purposes for which additional details are required, for example, ethnic origin and social class may be needed for some surveys.

PRACTICE RESEARCH DATABASE

This chapter is concerned with the collection of data from primary care using standardised methods. In effect, disciplined recording of morbidity in this way enables the development of a practice research database.[8] The standardisation of methods for data capture facilitates aggregation of data from individual practices to provide regional and national epidemiological information but also permits individual practitioners to compare their own experience with that of the group. Presented here are a few practical tips on how such a high quality database can be achieved.

Direct or indirect entry

In some practices, the GPs enter the morbidity data (direct entry), in others, a computer clerk undertakes the task (indirect entry). If entry is to be made by a clerk, there must be a clear convention as to how the notes are kept and the clerk must be informed of the appropriate entry and its episode type. A useful convention involves the use of the diagnostic triangle as a prefix before the relevant entry in the notes. The episode type is also recorded by the doctor – the simple descriptive terms First (F), New (N) and Ongoing (O) have proved easy to use in the Weekly Returns Service.

It is commonly the case that practices choose to have mixed data entry procedures. Often a clerk enters data from home visits or data relevant to consultations provided by locums. Sometimes in a partnership, one doctor is unhappy using the computer and a clerk will enter data for him.

Diagnostic consistency

The considerable detail of the Read coding system gives each doctor the opportunity to record data using his or her own preferred terminology. This can present problems when different doctors see a patient during one episode of illness. It is important first to record the diagnostic precision at the highest level of diagnostic specificity. An illness may present as back pain. Examination may not permit a more precise term than 'low back pain', or 'sciatica' if there is characteristic radiation. These terms are entirely appropriate, but if subsequent radiological examination defines particular pathology, that should be entered as the description of the morbidity in future. Once a specific pathology has been identified as the cause of the problem, it is inappropriate to revert back to describing the illness in symptomatic terms. Consistency is also important and where an episode of illness has been defined using one label – for example low back pain – then it should not subsequently be allocated a different name (e.g. sciatica) unless it is considered that the condition has changed.

Diagnostic amendments

Where there is a clear change of diagnosis, the entry should be amended. The principle to be adopted is that amendment should be made where the original information is incorrect. An entry of appendicitis is wrong if the patient turned out to have pelvic inflammatory disease. An entry of acute bronchitis is not wrong if later the patient was found to have cancer of the bronchus. Bronchial cancer often presents as an unresolved episode of bronchitis. Routine disciplines need to be established whereby amendments are shown in the patient's medical records in a clear and consistent way.

Comprehensiveness of recording

This heading provides opportunity to emphasise the importance of the decision as to what is to be recorded. It is preferable to record a small amount of data consistently than attempt to record a large amount and fail to record it consistently.

COMBINING PRACTICE DATA

Data collected in ways outlined here have been used in national morbidity surveys and as part of the continuous monitoring programme in the sentinel practice network of the RCGP. In the annual report of the Birmingham Research Unit for 1996,[9] we have published a series of graphs comparing disease incidence in 1996 with that obtained by averaging the results for the previous 10 years. This is of both epidemiological interest and also of practical value for general practitioners in the understanding of seasonal variation in illness.

A participating general practitioner viewpoint

Norman Smith

Providing information for the Weekly Returns Service has become a way of life within our practice. In 1977, I started a new practice in the last major overspill development in the Midlands. It was an inner city practice, albeit in a semi-rural area. Prior to this, I had been in a health centre in Birmingham and had become aware of the Research Unit through Douglas Fleming. I remember well a visit to Robin Pinsent's practice in Handsworth, Birmingham in the late 1960s where I first saw the old College 'L' sheet and 'E' book in action. It was a revelation to see such organisation of information, especially as the records in the practice that I had recently joined were practically non-existent. It brought back memories of Derbyshire House in Manchester where, as a medical student, I was first introduced to the Lloyd George record system by Henry Ashworth, my GP tutor who often spoke of the 'mass of irretrievable information' sitting in the envelope.

Starting from a zero list in 1977 enabled me to generate a new A4 record system specially designed to make the information in the records more accessible, but it was in 1983 that, along with three other practices, we were able to start logging all patient contacts on computer, together with the consultation/episode code (F, N, O). We chose indirect entry as a means of easing the new discipline into the team and we have continued with this ever since.

Continuous recording makes two major demands on the doctor. The first is to be as accurate as possible in labelling the patient contact. The second is to be consistent and make sure that every contact is recorded. The input clerk has to be able to reject information and return to the GP if the correct entry code is not clear. The prospect of having a pile of notes returned certainly concentrated the mind in the early days and it is now rare for queries to be raised.

Audits of the accuracy of the levels of recording showed that we were achieving a high degree of consistency and it gives a feeling of satisfaction to contribute to the Weekly Returns Service, especially each time we receive the newsletter and the annual report.

A participating doctor's view of the Weekly Returns Service

Andy Ross

BACKGROUND

In 1985, I joined a practice which had been part of the Weekly Returns Service for several years. Here I have summarised, under different subheadings, what I feel I have gained from being a partner in a practice attached to the WRS.

THE CONSULTATION

First, my record-keeping became more focused. Gone were the encounters where records simply indicated a collection of jumbled symptoms with none of them marked as being key. I was forced to consider what problems were covered in the consultation and whether or not they were a manifestation of many diagnoses or just one, for example, anxiety. In addition, the need to assign an episode type to problems resulted in an inherent requirement to consider whether the patient had presented with the same problem previously.

As a result, my consultations with patients improved. Constantly questioning what each consultation was about led to a more critical appraisal of the diagnostic process. The use of symptom terms, such as low back pain or non-specific abdominal pain, as a diagnosis helped me not to assign a disease label at too early a stage. I recognised that labels help, but it is of course important to get them right.

Understanding period prevalence

Access to our practice morbidity database helped me understand the true dynamic nature of many illnesses. On our practice list at least 1100 patients have been seen with asthma at any time, but only half of these in the last year. If asked, 'How many asthmatics are there in your practice?', any reply has to be encased in a period prevalence. This factor was not appreciated by our health authority collecting data for annual reports.

Practice-based audit

In latter years I have greatly valued our computerised morbidity database for carrying out audit within the practice. I have carried out audits of the process of patient care, being readily able to identify patients with specific diseases. An audit of the management of urinary tract infection (UTI) in children demonstrates just how useful a single practice database can be.

In 1994, a search was made of our computer records to identify all children with a diagnosis of UTI in the preceding 3 years. The practice list size was 10 500. Ninety-three per cent of children initially thought to have a UTI had an MSU taken. In the few instances where an MSU was not done, clear follow-up arrangements were recorded in the notes.

The audit showed a 3-year prevalence of a proven UTI of 39/1238 (3.2%) in girls and 6/1277 (0.5%) in boys (1.8% overall). Of 42 children, 32 (76%) with first-proven or equivocal UTIs were referred to see a consultant. Of the 10 children (all girls) who were not referred, 9 had follow-up urine samples sent for MSU. All children not referred, except one, were aged over 5 years.

Of the 32 children referred to a consultant, 27 had an ultrasound scan and 5 had an ultrasound scan and a micturating cystourethrogram. Investigations were normal in 31 out of the 32 children referred. One girl aged 8 years at the time of the first UTI was found to have ureteric reflux.

The sample size turned out to be as large as that in many studies previously published in medical journals. The number of proven UTIs detected was higher than in most studies.

Three main findings emerged. First, that we were managing children suspected of having a UTI appropriately in the practice. Second, the low rate of abnormalities found really brought home the message that tests have to be targeted at the right population. Around the time of the audit it was still debated as to whether all children with a proven UTI should have a micturating cystourethrogram or an intravenous urogram. This would mean every girl in the country having at least a 10% lifetime chance of undergoing such a procedure, clearly a questionable policy. Third, the need for consultant referral in every case was also dubious.

I am pleased to report that we now have direct access to ultrasound of the urinary tract at our local hospital.

STUDENT TEACHING

Over the past two years medical students from Birmingham University seconded to the practice as part of their general practice attachment are asked by the Department of General Practice to carry out audits during their time with us. Our morbidity database allows us to readily identify patients with a whole range of conditions e.g. epilepsy, diabetes, ischaemic heart disease, stroke, rheumatoid arthritis, myocardial infarction, etc. The students can literally be asked 'Which disease are you particularly interested in?' or 'Which condition would you like to base your audit on?'.

FEEDBACK

Finally, my practice receives considerable feedback on how rates of diseases in our practice compare to others. We are sent a quarterly newsletter which keeps us abreast of topical issues, such as influenza activity, trends in infectious diseases, studies carried out at the Research Unit, IT developments and many more subjects.

REFERENCES

1. CGP (1954) *The College of General Practitioners Second Annual Report.* Records and Statistics Unit and Research Advisory Service, p. 24.

2. Logan WPD and Cushion AA (1958) Studies on medical and population subjects No.14. *Morbidity Statistics from General Practice*, vol.I–III (General). HMSO, London.

3. Research Unit of the Royal College of General Practitioners (1971) Diagnostic index. *Journal of the Royal College of General Practitioners.* **21**: 609.

4. Fleming DM, Norbury CA and Crombie DL (1991) *Annual and Seasonal Variation in the Incidence of Common Diseases.* Occasional Paper 53. Royal College of General Practitioners, London.

5. Read JD and Benson TJR (1986) Comprehensive coding. *British Journal of Health Care Computing.* **3**: 22–5.

6. Pinsent RJFH (1968) The evolving age/sex register. *Journal of the Royal College of General Practitioners.* **16**: 127–34.

7. Office of Population Censuses & Surveys (1995*) Morbidity Statistics from General Practice. Fourth National Study 1991–1992.* (eds A. McCormick, D. Fleming and J. Charlton) Series MB5 no.3. HMSO, London.

8. Fleming DM and Fullarton J (1993*) The Application of a General Practice Database to Pharmaco-epidemiology.* Occasional Paper 62. RCGP, London.

9. Weekly Returns Service Report for 1996 prepared by the Birmingham Research Unit of the Royal College of General Practitioners June 1997.

7

The RCGP Centre for Primary Care Research and Epidemiology

Philip Hannaford

THE OPPORTUNITY FOR EPIDEMIOLOGICAL RESEARCH

The central position of the primary care team within the NHS provides an important opportunity to undertake long-term epidemiological research. Almost everyone living in the UK is registered with a named general practitioner who contracts to provide primary care services. Each practice, therefore, cares for a defined population from which individuals with particular characteristics can be identified and recruited for research purposes. These characteristics might include the existence of a medical condition such as diabetes or hypertension, use of a particular service or receipt of a specified treatment. The practice list also facilitates the identification of individuals without the chosen characteristic, so that a suitable comparison group can be assembled. The effort needed to identify potential subjects for a study has been reduced in recent years by the widespread computerisation of general practices.

The gatekeeper role of the GP means that few patients are seen by colleagues in the secondary or tertiary care sector without referral from a GP. This is especially so in the era of fundholding and locality-based commissioning of services. The usual feedback of information about the outcome of the hospital visit enables practices to compile comprehensive records of a person's use of medical services. The transfer of these records from the old practice to the new one when a patient moves helps ensure that the records contain details of the main medical events occurring during a person's life.

The quality and comprehensiveness of the medical records held by the primary care team is constantly being improved. This is partly because of a growing awareness of the medicolegal importance of having complete and accurate medical records. It also reflects recent trends towards giving the primary care team a central role in the coordination of preventive services, such as childhood immunisation programmes, the detection of hypertension and screening for cervical and breast cancer. A further impetus has been the increasing use of computers in the consultation room to record information about presenting symptoms, examination findings, diagnoses, information likely to be useful in future consultations (such as smoking and drinking habits), medical procedures provided and prescriptions issued.

THE SUCCESSFUL EXPLOITATION OF THIS OPPORTUNITY

For nearly 30 years, the Royal College of General Practitioners' (RCGP) Centre for Primary Care Research and Epidemiology (formerly the RCGP Manchester Research Unit) has successfully exploited the opportunity provided by general practice to undertake epidemiological research. A particular strength of the Centre is its ability to recruit hundreds of GPs willing to provide, often on an unpaid basis, comprehensive patient-specific data for extended periods of time. By asking a large number of practitioners (or their staff) to each supply information about a comparatively small number of patients, the workload of the individual practitioner is kept small. The use of simple data collection forms, with the minimum of rules for their completion, also reduces the workload. By successfully coordinating this collective effort, the Centre manages to accumulate the vast quantities of data required for its research.

All of the Centre's senior scientific staff has experience of general practice. Indeed, the Manchester Research Unit's first director, Dr Clifford Kay, combined an internationally recognised research career with that of a busy GP for more than 25 years. This involvement with general practice helps to ensure that the Centre's work is relevant to the primary care team. It also means that there is a strong understanding of the strengths and weaknesses of data collected from general practice, thereby avoiding the erroneous interpretation of such information.

ORAL CONTRACEPTION STUDY

The Centre was established in 1968 to conduct the Oral Contraception Study, an investigation which illustrates many of the principles employed in the subsequent studies.

By the mid-1960s, a rapidly increasing number of women were using oral contraceptives. It was recognized, however, that little was known about the health effects of these preparations especially in the long term. New studies were needed, not only to confirm or refute problems already thought to be associated with the use of oral contraception, but also to detect effects not previously suspected. A cohort study which collected information about a variety of health outcomes represented the most efficient way of determining the overall risks and benefits associated with the use of oral contraception. Furthermore, since this type of study involves the calculation of disease incidence rates, information would become available about the absolute risks (or benefits) associated with the use of oral contraception, enabling women and their advisors to put any effects into perspective. Basing a new cohort study in general practice offered two distinct advantages. First, the opportunity to collect information about the wide range of medical problems presented to the GP, including those that rarely result in referral to hospital. Second, the possibility of making the study large enough to permit detailed examination of the relationship between uncommon disease and the use of the Pill.

During a 14-month period starting in May 1968, 1400 GPs throughout the UK recruited 23 000 women who were using oral contraceptives and a similar number who had never done so.[1] All of the women were married or living as married, their average age was 29 years and most were Caucasian. Information collected at recruitment included details of any previous use of oral contraception, the occupation of the woman's husband (to determine her social class), the woman's smoking habits, parity and significant past medical history. Patient confidentiality was maintained by allocating each woman a unique study number, the key to which only the GP held; all correspondence between the Centre and the doctor has used this study number.

At 6-monthly intervals since recruitment, participating doctors have supplied details of any: hormonal preparations prescribed (initially oral contraceptives but more recently hormone replacement therapies), pregnancies and their outcome, surgery and the reason for it, all new episodes of illness reported to the GP and, when appropriate, date and cause of death. Diagnostic criteria have not been provided for the GPs. In some cases, the reported diagnoses have been those made by the participating GP or another member of the primary care team. In others, the participating doctors will have simply reported the opinion of hospital colleagues who may have had access to the results of investigations, operation notes or post-mortem findings. Serious conditions which are more likely to result in referral to hospital, such as cancers or cardiovascular events, have a higher proportion of reports based on this supplementary information than less serious conditions which are managed more frequently in the community. As well as having access to the opinion of hospital colleagues, the GPs in the study benefit from observing their patients over a prolonged period of time. Diagnoses which are initially uncertain may become clearer later. Indeed, the study often needs to revise its recorded diagnoses as additional information becomes available. In general, the study's findings have been consistent with those from other studies, including those which used specific diagnostic criteria.

Nearly three-quarters of the cohort has now been lost to GP follow-up, mainly because of the women leaving the recruiting practice. During the early years of the study attempts were made to trace women to their new practice to seek its help with the follow-up. Unfortunately, the procedure met with only limited success and so had to be abandoned. No data collected for the study, however, is wasted, since all women contribute to the database up to the date they leave the study. In addition, during the late 1970s, 75% of the cohort was flagged at the NHS Central Registries in Southport and Edinburgh. This means that the Centre is notified of any deaths or cancer registrations occurring in these women, even among those no longer under GP observation. (The remaining 25% of women could not be flagged because they, or their GP, had already left the study when the flagging procedure took place.)

So far, the study has accumulated more than 550 000 woman-years of observation making it one of the largest detailed studies of oral contraception in the world. It was among the first to show that the risk of cardiovascular disease among Pill users who smoke is much higher than that among users who do not smoke, especially in older women.[2,3] These findings continue to influence clinical practice. The study was the first to demonstrate that the risk of hypertension[4] and arterial disease[5] is related to the progestogen content of the Pill. Evidence from the study that users of combined oral contraceptives may have a lower risk of rheumatoid arthritis[6] led to a flurry of new studies around the world investigating this unexpected finding. A recent analysis of the database to examine the long-term cardiovascular sequelae of toxaemia of pregnancy (now generally referred to as pre-eclampsia) indicated that women with a history of this condition have higher risks of hypertension, myocardial infarction, other forms of ischaemic heart disease, venous thromboembolic disease and possibly stroke than women without such a history.[7] This finding has led to the launch of a new study, the Aberdeen Study of Cardiovascular Health in Women, which will investigate further this intriguing relationship.

ATTITUDES TO PREGNANCY STUDY

The rising number of women having an induced abortion during the early 1970s led to questions being raised in Parliament regarding the safety of this procedure. Aware of the success of the Oral Contraception Study, the Department of Health approached the RCGP to see whether it could undertake a similar observational study of the health effects of induced abortion. This led to the euphemistically titled Attitudes to Pregnancy Study, a collaborative effort between the RCGP and the Royal College of Obstetricians and Gynaecologists. The study was coordinated by the Manchester Research Unit under the supervision of its former deputy director, Dr Peter Frank.

Between 1976 and 1978, 1509 GPs in England, Scotland and Wales recruited about 7000 women who had an induced abortion and 7000 women who presented with an unplanned pregnancy who did not request a termination of pregnancy.[8] Baseline information collected included the woman's age, marital status, smoking habits, age at completion of full-time education (used to measure social status), and previous medical, psychiatric and obstetric history. Nearly 800 gynaecologists working in both the NHS and the private sector provided details of the consultation during which the abortion request was considered, and if performed, gave details of the operation and its early complications. The GPs subsequently supplied, for up to ten years, information about any new pregnancies and their outcome, reported morbidities and, when appropriate, cause of death.

The study was able to assess the effects of induced abortion on short-term health,[9] future fertility,[10] subsequent pregnancies[11] and psychiatric health.[12] In general, the results were reassuring, with few associations observed either in the short or long term. Given the sensitive nature of the operation, a major strength of the study was its ability to maintain patient confidentiality by using the system of allocating a special study number developed for the Oral Contraception Study. Indeed, in a pilot survey, nearly half the women who had an induced abortion said they would refuse to participate in a study if they could not remain anonymous.

OTHER WORK

The Centre's expertise in providing the logistic support needed to undertake large-scale studies has been used successfully in a number of other studies. The RCGP Myocardial Infarction Study was an 18-month investigation of the safety and feasibility of the domiciliary use of anistreplase by GPs.[13] The Evaluation of Take Care project assessed whether the introduction of a commercially sponsored education programme improved the ability of GPs to recognise psychological illness.[14] The Wythenshawe Community Asthma Project is a continuing longitudinal study of the natural history of respiratory symptoms affecting patients from two practices in South Manchester, UK.[15] The project will also examine the costs associated with treating asthma.

Less successful was the Centre's involvement in the early 1990s in the European Investigation of Cancer (EPIC), a European-wide prospective study of the relationship between diet and cancer. In conjunction with the Imperial Cancer Research Fund's (ICRF) Cancer Epidemiology Unit in Oxford, UK, the Centre agreed to be responsible for recruiting 50 000 middle-aged men and women via GPs working throughout the UK. Participation in EPIC also appeared to provide a useful opportunity to investigate the long-term effects of hormone replacement therapy. The study was launched in Scotland with subsequent extensions into northern England. To ease administration of the study, women were to be recruited first; participating practices being asked to recruit two users and two non-users of hormone replacement therapy each month. The recruitment procedure, however, was far from simple. The doctors needed to identify suitable patients during routine consultations, obtain written informed consent, complete a complicated recruitment form and take a blood sample for dispatch to a central laboratory in Cambridge. The women also had to complete a detailed food frequency questionnaire and a food diary. Not surprisingly, few doctors felt able to commit time to the study even though many felt that the research questions were important. The poor recruitment rates meant that recruitment via the GP had to be abandoned. More successful, alternative methods of recruitment have now been established; these are now being coordinated by the ICRF Unit in Oxford.

Several hard but important lessons were learnt during the Centre's involvement in EPIC. First, it is vital to remember the realities of life in a busy general practice; wherever possible simplify, simplify and simplify again the recruitment procedures. In particular, do not overcomplicate matters by trying to answer too many research questions at the same time. Second, if we intend to ask members of the primary care team to help us in our research, we must actively seek (and obtain) some way of compensating them for their work. Alternatively we must put research personnel into practices to undertake the work. Third, although we piloted the recruitment procedures for EPIC, these pilot studies were clearly not extensive enough to give us a reliable picture of likely recruitment in the main study.

FUTURE DEVELOPMENTS

In September 1997, the RCGP Manchester Research Unit was relocated to RCGP Centre of Primary Care Research and Epidemiology within the Department of General Practice and Primary Care at the University of Aberdeen. The Centre is the new home for the valuable datasets accumulated in Manchester. These databases offer the opportunity to gain new insights into the aetiology of many diseases, particularly those affecting women.

Over the years, the Centre's research interests have broadened from the effects of specific medical interventions to more general issues that come under the heading of primary care epidemiology. Thus, the Centre is now interested in issues such as the measurement of the frequency of disease and symptoms recorded by the primary care team or reported by patients in the community; the factors likely to influence the onset of these diseases or symptoms; the long-term impact of these problems on subsequent health; and the appropriate role of screening for disease in the primary care setting. The relocation of the Centre to Aberdeen provides easier access to colleagues with recognized expertise in the measurement of symptoms and health outcomes, health economics and molecular science; skills which complement those already within the Centre and which are likely to be needed in future research projects. The development of new multidisciplinary, collaborative studies will ensure that the Centre continues to provide the primary care team with some of the information that it needs to practise evidence-based medicine.

REFERENCES

1. Royal College of General Practitioners (1974) *Oral Contraceptives and Health*. Pitman Medical Publishing, Tunbridge Wells.

2. Royal College of General Practitioners' Oral Contraception Study (1977) Mortality among oral contraceptive users. *Lancet*. **ii**: 727–31.

3. Royal College of General Practitioners' Oral Contraception Study (1983) Incidence of arterial disease among oral contraceptive users. *Journal of the Royal College of General Practitioners*. **33**: 75–82.

4. Royal College of General Practitioners' Oral Contraception Study (1977) Effect on hypertension and benign breast disease of progestogen component in combined oral contraceptives. *Lancet*. **i**: 624.

5. Kay CR (1982) Progestogens and arterial disease – evidence from the Royal College of General Practitioners' study. *American Journal of Obstetrics and Gynaecology*. **142**: 762–5.

6. Royal College of General Practitioners' Oral Contraception Study (1978) Reduction in the incidence of rheumatoid arthritis associated with oral contraceptives. *Lancet*. **i**: 569–71.

7. Hannaford P, Ferry S and Hirsch S (1997) Cardiovascular sequelae of toxaemia of pregnancy. *Heart*. **77**: 154–8.

8. Kay CR and Frank PI (1981) Characteristics of women recruited to a long-term study of the sequelae of induced abortion. *Journal of the Royal College of General Practitioners*. **31**: 473–7.

9. Joint Study of the Royal College of General Practitioners and the Royal College of Obstetricians and Gynaecologists (1985) Induced abortion operations and their early sequelae. *Journal of the Royal College of General Practitioners*. **35**: 175–80.

10. Frank P, McNamee R, Hannaford PC *et al.* (1993) The effect of induced abortion on subsequent fertility. *British Journal of Obstetrics and Gynaecology*. **100**: 575–80.

11. Frank PI, McNamee R, Hannaford PC *et al.* (1991) The effect of induced abortion on subsequent pregnancy outcome. *British Journal of Obstetrics and Gynaecology*. **98**: 1015–24.

12. Gilchrist AC, Hannaford PC, Frank P *et al.* (1995) Termination of pregnancy and psychiatric morbidity. *British Journal of Psychiatry*. **167**: 243–8.

13. Hannaford P, Vincent R, Ferry S *et al.* (1995) Assessment of the practicality and safety of thrombolysis with anistreplase given by general practitioners. *British Journal of General Practice*. **45**: 175–9.

14. Hannaford PC, Thompson C and Simpson M (1996) Evaluation of an educational programme to improve the recognition of psychological illness by general practitioners. *British Journal of General Practice.* **46**: 333–7.

15. Frank P, Ferry S, Moorhead T *et al.* (1996) Use of a postal questionnaire to estimate the likely under-diagnosis of asthma-like illness in adults. *British Journal of General Practice.* **46**: 295–7.

8

How to do higher degrees in primary care

Tony Avery, Yvonne Carter and Amanda Howe

Most of the knowledge and much of the genius of the research worker lie behind his selection of what is worth observing. It is a crucial choice, often determining the success or failure of months of work, often differentiating the brilliant discoverer from the ... plodder.

Alan Gregg[1]

The conventional picture of the research worker is that of a rather austere man in a white coat with a background of complicated glassware. My idea of a research worker, on the other hand, is a man who brushes his teeth on the left side of his mouth only so as to use the other side as a control and see if tooth brushing has any effect on the incidence of caries.

Sir Robert Platt[2]

INTRODUCTION

Research opportunities for primary care workers have increased dramatically over recent years, paralleled by expansion in research capacity through university departments of primary care, the development of research networks,[3] and funding for research training[4] and infrastructure.[5, 6] Although some of these initiatives are at an early stage and their impact is as yet unclear,[7] these developments mean that an increasing number of primary care workers are considering carrying out higher degrees. This chapter will describe the options available to primary care workers and will offer a framework from our own experience to consider the advantages and disadvantages of undertaking a higher degree.

BACKGROUND

While research opportunities have increased recently, there is still a paucity of higher degrees among primary care staff compared with many other groups of health professionals. For example, between 1973 and 1988 only 50 doctorates of medicine in the British Isles came from general practice (accounting for just 1.6% of all successful MD theses).[8]

Concern has been raised about underdevelopment of research capacity in primary care. While the main way of tackling this problem will involve the provision of adequate resources,[4, 5] it has been suggested that the best way to produce good researchers in general practice is to encourage individuals to 'accept the challenge of writing a PhD or an MD thesis'.[8] We would agree with this, and suggest that by encouraging primary care workers to carry out higher degrees there will be the following important benefits to our disciplines:

- an increase in quality research that will help us in our professional practices
- an increase in the status of primary healthcare professionals
- an increase in intellectual rigour developed as a consequence of in-depth academic study
- an increase in academic stimulation to encourage intellectual enquiry.

The following sections will example some of the 'why, what and how' of undertaking higher degrees from primary care.

WHY DO A HIGHER DEGREE?

There are a number of reasons for undertaking a higher degree. In some cases it may be a means to an end. For example, any primary care worker hoping to have a career in an academic discipline is increasingly likely to need a higher degree. In other cases, the research may be an end in itself with a professional wishing to 'satisfy a curiosity'[8] and enjoying the intellectual challenge of the research process. Whatever the reason for undertaking a higher degree, those who do so will gain an exceptional intellectual training in the process, including:

- the ability to locate, critique and distil academic literature
- the systematic storage, recall and organisation of material
- the use of information technology for many inter-related purposes
- a detailed knowledge of research methodology

- a detailed knowledge of data analysis, using quantitative and/or qualitative methods
- understanding the practicalities of research, including ethical issues, relationships with research colleagues and subjects, managing resources and systematic planning
- learning from peer review and external assessment.

Implicit in this list is a new level of personal and professional development, which might include:

- the ability to critique and refine one's own work
- the ability to plan and carry through a long-term project
- time and resource management
- new insights into the strengths and weaknesses of one's intellect
- new insights into the strengths and weaknesses of one's own character
- an appreciation of both the enjoyment and sheer hard work involved in delivering new knowledge.

Whether primary care staff are inspired to take up the opportunity of a higher degree may depend not only on their own ambitions, but also on whether they are exposed to role models who may inspire them towards this end. It may depend on the ethos of their working setting; that is, whether there is an active local culture of primary care research. Finally, it may depend on whether opportunities are created whereby staff can move from the idea of doing a higher degree to making it a reality.

WHO DOES HIGHER DEGREES?

Several surveys have been performed on general practitioners with higher degrees.[8–10] These surveys showed that the number of higher degrees averaged just three per year between 1973 and 1988 compared with five per year in the previous 15 years. Fortunately the numbers of successful MD theses coming from general practice has increased in the 1990s,[11] and this trend looks likely to continue.

While one would expect academic general practitioners to take up higher degrees, it is important to note that between 1973 and 1988 two-thirds of successful MD theses came from GPs who did not have a university appointment.[8] This suggests that support for higher degrees needs to extend beyond university departments. We also know that a similar expansion is occurring within nursing. With increased funding for primary care research, we hope that opportunities will improve for *all* professionals involved in primary care to take up the challenge of completing a higher degree.

WHAT'S INVOLVED IN DOING A HIGHER DEGREE?

Universities have traditionally offered graduates the opportunity to submit either a Masters in Philosophy (MPhil) or a Doctor of Philosophy (PhD) degree through their own original research, the former being both an end point in itself and a stage to the latter. Many such degrees now require a formal research training programme in the first year, which might include material on research methods. However, there is an expectation that the majority of time will be spent on the candidate's own work. Medical candidates have the option of a Doctorate of Medicine (DM or MD) degree. Although many candidates will take longer, the relative full-time commitments and equivalent depth of work for these higher degrees are one year for an MPhil, two for an MD and three for a PhD.

The regulations for higher research degrees vary from one university to another and you are strongly advised to check both written requirements and experience of colleagues at an early stage. In particular, MD candidates may have to register with their university of origin unless they hold a post at another university. Information on regulations for higher degrees may be obtained from the graduate office of a university. These regulations are likely to advise on:

- eligibility for registration
- how to register for a higher degree
- fees
- the minimum and maximum times permissible between registration and submission of the higher degree
- arrangements for supervision
- the format in which the higher degree should be submitted
- how the higher degree will be examined.

To carry out a higher degree one needs to:

- identify one or more research questions to which the answer is not yet known
- search the literature for all relevant background
- refine the research questions into an answerable form
- design studies that are capable of answering the questions (rooted in the literature, with appropriate methods and samples)
- carry out the research
- analyse the findings
- write up the research, including detailed discussion
- submit a thesis for examination.

In terms of *process*, a successful higher degree is likely to require:

- much personal time, energy and commitment
- support and forbearance from family and colleagues
- access to relevant literature (both electronically and hard copy)
- some kind of mentoring or formal supervision
- advice and training in research methods

- statistical advice
- access to information technology
- time to collect and collate data, *or* help from a research assistant
- money – for time out, fees, materials and staff assistance.

Further information and advice on carrying out a higher degree is available from other sources.[12]

HOW CAN I GET RESOURCES FOR DOING A HIGHER DEGREE?

The three inter-related resource requirements for higher degrees (time out, fees and materials, staff assistance) all have potential costs attached. For most NHS staff, by far the greatest cost will be buying their time out of the practice. Sources of funding worth exploring are:

- Professional study leave: GPs can be granted prolonged study leave by the NHS Executive if they fulfil the requirements of the 'Red Book'.[13]
- Research grants: applications can be submitted for funding of particular projects, for example to the Scientific Foundation Board of the Royal College of General Practitioners, the Department of Health and various charities. However, these grants are competitive and novice researchers may struggle to secure funding with their preliminary efforts at research design.
- Support for research infrastructure: practices can apply for this through the Culyer initiative.
- The Royal Colleges and local academic bodies may have specific grants, scholarships and fellowships available for those seeking a research training.
- Regional offices and the research councils (MRC and ESRC) may also be able to help.

Many universities and regions have some sort of research advisory service, and some will fund initial research methods training. Access to information on registration, information technology, libraries, supervision and statistical advice may be sought via local academic units of general practice, primary care or nursing. These units may also be able to advise on additional sources of funding. Additional staff time to support primary care researchers may also be available from the local academic and NHS providers. This is particularly true if an individual project is part of another larger-scale proposal, or if the practice itself has attracted research funding through which staff can be temporarily employed.

Even with access to the resources outlined above, candidates for higher degrees often have to pay for:

- registration of the higher degree
- IT for use at home
- printing and binding of the thesis (several copies may be required).

Undertaking a higher degree may require considerable financial resources. While candidates may be able to obtain external funding and support, they need to be aware that there is likely to be a personal financial cost.

WHAT ARE THE OUTCOMES OF DOING A HIGHER DEGREE?

There are a number of potential outcomes from doing a higher degree. At a personal level, the successful candidate is likely to have a sense of achievement, a new intellectual approach to practice and a new sphere of future activity. Professionally, there will be kudos, letters after the name, potential for publications and further research,[8] and opportunities for promotion. Altruistically, they will now be able to supervise and assist others in their research efforts, and can be confident that they have contributed to the body of professional knowledge.

There can, however, be negative outcomes, and these must be taken into account. The higher degree candidate must make a realistic assessment of their own intellectual and material capabilities before embarking on a prolonged and arduous task (local advice may be helpful here). Many higher degrees remain uncompleted, and this may represent personal disappointment and wasted resources. The energies required will be taken out of some alternative project (in the practice or at home), and so the cost-benefits must be considered. The knowledge gained is deep rather than wide, and will have limited applicability to the requirements of daily clinical practice. Finally, the findings of a study may not be headline news and this may be disheartening, albeit not likely to cause failure of the degree.

IN CONCLUSION

This section has presented some of the basic 'nuts and bolts' of higher degrees to help the reader consider whether this option might be for them. The next section presents a more personal view of our experiences as candidates, which we hope will aid you further in developing your thinking.

Higher degrees in primary care: some experiences from the front line

Tony Avery

I became interested in primary care research when studying for my MRCGP examination. I was struck by the potential for improving patient care through the implementation of research finding and decided on a career in academic general practice. On joining the Department of General Practice at Nottingham I felt that carrying out a higher degree would be a good way of developing my research skills. Also, it was made clear that a higher degree was essential for career progression. I had a number of ideas for research projects and one of these involved evaluating the impact of the introduction of prescribing formularies in general practice. With one of the senior lecturers, I obtained funding for this research and was given the opportunity to manage the project under supervision. Carrying out this project gave me ideas for further related research and I managed to obtain funding for a research assistant to help carry out these studies. In thinking about my higher degree it gradually became clear that there was a consistent thread running throughout the studies and this allowed me to piece them together into a coherent whole.

This may sound fairly straightforward. However, it is worth noting that I could not have predicted the direction of my studies from the outset. The development of my ideas was an evolving process and the direction that I took was partly related to the funding opportunities available. As an academic general practitioner I had time to carry out my research and I was helped by having the support of research assistants, a statistician and my supervisor. However, it still involved a lot of hard work. The major challenge for me came at the writing up stage. I was already working long hours with research, teaching, clinical and administrative duties. How could I find the time to write up the thesis?

With the support of the department I was relieved of some teaching and administrative responsibilities, and I was given some funding to take a day a week out of my practice for five months. This created a defined period to try and complete the thesis. During this time I worked on the thesis for two weekdays per week, for at least a day each weekend and nearly every evening. It felt like climbing a very big mountain and I often had to force myself back to the computer after any sort of break. Eventually, bit by bit, the thesis came together and I was able to complete it within my self-imposed deadline. I feel pleased with the result, although I know that it could have been better if I had given myself more time. However, this would have meant even greater disruption to my personal and family life and I decided to settle on a 'good enough' thesis.

Since completing my higher degree I have felt a number of benefits. These include:

- an improvement in my critical ability to appraise and distil literature
- an improvement in my research skills
- a greater appreciation of the importance of using rigorous research methods and of scientific enquiry
- a boost to my self-esteem: it feels good to have succeeded in completing a doctorate of medicine.

What key messages do I have for anyone contemplating a higher degree? First, you must choose a topic that interests you. Second, it is essential to have adequate training in research methods. Third, supervision (including critical appraisal) of your work is important. Finally, make sure that you leave some quality time for yourself and your family: you all deserve it.

Yvonne Carter

The child is burned! I never hear that announcement without a shudder, for it has opened the portals to a long avenue of pain and distress, an avenue that may lead to an age-long disfigurement and too often, by shorter ways, to the tragedy of death. Let us take counsel together about it. Wherein are its dangers? What are its risks? How can disaster be mitigated or avoided?

Sir John Fraser[14]

The quotation above poignantly describes how I became interested in studying accidents in children. During my vocational training I spent six months as a senior house officer in the accident and emergency department of Alder Hey Children's Hospital in Liverpool. During that time I still recall a 'critical incident' when a whole family was involved in a serious house fire. The memory of that day in casualty has remained with me.

Accidents are the leading cause of death in pre-school children in the UK and historically accidents *per se* had been little researched in general practice. When choosing the topic for my thesis I needed to consider if it was interesting, important, common, relevant and achievable. I felt that childhood accidents fulfilled all the criteria. My MD thesis examined the relative roles of education, environmental modification and legislation in child accident prevention. The thesis described a number of small studies with a common theme of childhood accidents in the same district. If your university regulations allow I cannot overemphasise the importance of publishing and presenting your work as you go. As well as receiving peer-reviewed feedback on your work, you will grow in confidence and will be able to impress your examiners with your reprints.

Box 8.1

- Think about it
- Talk about it
- Read about it
- Do it!
- Publish as you go

Identifying and addressing my personal training needs included attendance at three courses: epidemiology for clinicians in Southampton, research methods at St George's and a computing course in Manchester. It was also important to identify and contact key informants in the field. For accidents this involved making contact with individuals and organisations as well as attending some topic specific meetings and workshops.

To set the study in context, I reviewed the literature describing the importance and variations that occur in childhood accidents and the various attempts to explain them. A developmental approach is useful in understanding the causes of injury and in planning prevention. The kind of events in which a child is likely to be injured depend on the child's abilities and where, how and with whom the child spends time, all of which change as the child grows and matures. The study began with an observation that accidents in young children are common, that few are treated initially by the general practitioner and that accidents seem to occur more commonly when families are under stress. This observation proved to be a good starting point for the study.

My MD thesis was designed to encourage family doctors, health visitors and teachers to make child accident prevention a higher priority in their professional work. It was the result of three years' work from July 1990 to August 1993. During this time I continued to work as a 26-hour principal in North Staffordshire and for the first two years had two sessions of protected time each week funded through an RCGP Research Training Fellowship. During that time I was an honorary research fellow at Keele University. In the final year of the thesis I had a part-time sessional appointment as a senior lecturer at the University of Birmingham. I sacrificed time for my family and for me and had no extended study leave. I remember spending a large part of a two-week summer holiday printing four copies of the thesis and delivering it to the binders!

The opportunity to leave a full-time principal post in Liverpool after three years and move to the Midlands when my husband took up his first consultant post gave me the opportunity to reflect on what I really wanted to do with my career. I had moved straight into a busy principal post on completing my trainee year without giving any thought to making time to do research. I had completed several small projects as a student and junior doctor and it was only when I was overwhelmed with a heavy clinical load that I missed the opportunity to do research. I had always wanted to successfully complete an MD since my days as an undergraduate and I suppose I had always intended to submit through my Alma Mater (St Mary's

Hospital Medical School in London). This I achieved with a local supervisor in Keele and a London supervisor who kept in touch by post and an annual face-to-face meeting.

I am now in the position of both supervising five MD theses (one by e-mail from Malaysia) and examining both MDs and PhDs. The quality of our work in primary care must be maintained at the same level as our professional colleagues from secondary care. In my role as Chairman of Research for the RCGP I am currently responsible for maintaining a directory of higher degrees in general practice and an extensive collection of theses is available for viewing from the library (remember to book first). Some excellent examples are ready to stimulate the imagination of what is possible from primary care.

Amanda Howe

I first considered the idea of doing a higher degree at my interview for a part-time lecturer post in the Department of General Practice in Sheffield in 1991. Until then, I had been an active junior partner for seven years, and a mum for four, so the desire to extend my commitments had only recently occurred to me. I had applied predominantly because I was interested in teaching, and had read all I could about medical education and curricular reform. The one surprise question was whether I had thought of doing an MD – the answer was clearly meant to be yes, but at the same time a light flashed up in my brain: 'now there's an idea'. It seems extraordinary that no one had ever offered this vision to me before, and indeed that I had not pursued it myself. I had many friends who were in hospital careers and had considered their research training a matter of routine. Why not GPs? Why not me?

Having been appointed, my interest was rapidly cultivated, and within a year I had taken three months of leave from my practice, failed to get a research grant, and nevertheless set up a project with fieldwork planned into the next year. My professor described doing an MD from a clinical base as 'a full-time hobby' – and he was right! Reading even half the literature I identified was more academic reading than I had done since taking membership, and rushing from my own practice to recruit GPs elsewhere made my own working day (and theirs) even longer than usual. Old habits of organising material and previous IT skills came in very useful, but the thoroughness and focus required for excellent intellectual endeavour was often missing as I struggled to stay awake poring over esoteric articles on somatisation.

The department was an unstinting source of support and resources: I was given regular supervision and free access to a research methods course. Study leave and some research assistant time were both paid for out of departmental moneys set aside for novice GP researchers. There were few other MD candidates, so I was without peer support, but the excellence of my supervision (not obligatory to MD candidates) was more than adequate compensation. My practice were also endlessly tolerant; having allowed me maternity leave, a further sabbatical in a total career of a potential 30 years may not seem excessive, but I was immensely impressed by their 'unconditional positive regard' for what was generally considered a rather unexciting cause (as in 'why don't you go trekking in Nepal instead?'). I was able to secure six months prolonged study leave to write up my thesis, which was barely long enough: I delivered it to the examinations office within 24 hours of my return to work, and less than four years from when the idea was first raised.

It is interesting to look back and ask three questions:

- what helped me to get through?
- what do I feel about the process in retrospect?
- if I had the choice, would I do a higher degree again?

I have already mentioned the considerable material and personal support offered to me by department and practice: if I include family support, three important elements for success are highlighted. A real interest in my subject matter and a growing enjoyment of the sifting and analysing of academic material captured my initial commitment. A clear expectation that I would succeed and that my achievement would matter both as a role model to others and in my own career was a personal pressure on me to believe in my ability and to struggle on. A growing sense of obligation and energies already invested by both myself and others made giving up halfway look unacceptable There was a certain detective streak in analysing the data, and seeing whether I could 'disprove the null hypothesis'. Writing up was greatly helped by having uninterrupted time to do it, though I often longed for real people to work with instead of words and figures. The end point deadline helped me to deliver.

It is difficult to be positive about the process, because my immediate memory is that it was often lonely, difficult and confusing. Many skills (particularly computing and statistics) were initially lacking, and I had to become used to delayed gratification and multiple reworking of data and text. I remember being shocked by the 'adult' relationship evoked by my supervisor, who made no attempt to mark my work or to fill gaps in knowledge. The sense that only I could tell if my arguments were 'right or wrong' was alarming, especially in the oral examination phase. I often asked myself why I was doing it, and found the reassurance of others hollow. The dogged determination required was considerable and the lifestyle unhealthy – hardly a balanced intellectual diet. Nevertheless there were moments of satisfaction – when the literature review structure popped into my head, when the intervention data came out positive, when I had the confidence to challenge my supervisor, when I argued my case in the viva and when I finally put on the silly hat and was awarded my degree.

Would I do it again? Yes, because I am no longer intellectually browned off, but get huge pleasure and stimulation out of many academic sources. Yes, because I now think and write differently. Yes, because I can now supervise others and see them grow in understanding and confidence. Yes, because I needed the qualification to gain a full-time academic post (it made all the difference to my chances of promotion, but I did not start out with this intention). No, if I wanted someone to provide structure or to get some variety in my studies (do a Masters). No, if I wanted to focus on clinical issues and stay as a full-time GP (for me, the MD was a step away rather than toward general practice). No, if I wanted to be loved rather than admired by my family. And no, if I had not had the space in my life to make such a full-time commitment to my own work.

The more important question, however, for the reader is not 'would I' but 'would *you* do a higher degree if you had the chance?'

REFERENCES

1. Gregg A (1941) *The Furtherance of Medical Research*. Elliots Books, Northford, CT, USA.

2. Platt R (1953) Opportunities for research in general practice. *BMJ*. **i**: 577–80.

3. Hungin APS (1995) *Research Networks in Primary Care in the UK: proceedings of a national conference on networks*. Northern Research Network, Stockton on Tees.

4. Mant D (1997) *National Working Group on R&D in Primary Care: final report*. NHS Executive, London.

5. Research & Development Task Force (1994) *Supporting Research & Development in the NHS*. A report to the Minister for health by a research & development task force chaired by Professor Anthony Culyer. HMSO, London.

6. NHS Executive (1997) *R&D Funding for NHS Providers*. NHSE, Leeds.

7. Carter YH (1997) Funding research in primary care: is Culyer the remedy? *British Journal of General Practice*. **47**: 543–4.

8. Williams WO (1990) A survey of doctorates by thesis among general practitioners in the British Isles from 1973 to 1988. *British Journal of General Practice*. **40**: 491–4.

9. Williams WO (1974) MD by thesis from general practice. *Journal of the Royal College of General Practitioners* **24**: 778–83.

10. Williams WO (1969) MD by thesis from general practice. *British Journal of Medical Education* **3**(3): 171–5.

11. Royal College of General Practitioners (1996) *Members Reference Book 1996*. RCGP, London.

12. Phillips EM and Pugh DS (1994) *How to Get a PhD*, 2nd edn. Open University, Milton Keynes.

13. Department of Health and Welsh Office (1996) *National Health Service General Medical Services. Statement of fees and allowances payable to general medical practitioners in England and Wales 1996 edition*. Department of Health, London.

14. Fraser J (1927) The treatment of burns in children. *BMJ*. **i**: 1089–92.

9

Taught Masters courses

Cathryn Thomas

Throughout the UK a number of university departments are offering taught courses which lead to a Masters degree. Most of these courses started in the 1980s and early 1990s in response to the need to train general practitioners and others working in primary care in research methods and appraisal skills, to improve the output of research from primary care.

A taught Masters course is often a good place to start for GPs, community nurses and others who have been out of an academic environment for some time. The content of the course is different at each institution but most are based around such ideas as: learning to think critically about day-to-day practice, appraisal of literature, research design and methodologies. Most also involve undertaking a piece of original research written up as a dissertation. The taught component of the course obviously offers the students the opportunity to learn from 'experts' much more than undertaking a PhD or MD does, but it also offers a structure which is reassuring to those who are tentative about whether they can cope with the workload and the intellectual effort. Courses are designed to support the learners while gradually encouraging independent work until the student is running their own project with occasional help from their supervisor.

For many the reason they embark on a taught course is not so much to do with a burning desire to learn about research – although that is certainly true for some – as with a desire to broaden their horizons. Often the routine of general practice and primary care lacks stimulation after a while and students are seeking a challenge. When they become immersed in the course they frequently 'get the research bug' and there is no stopping them. The support and camaraderie of the group is a vital part of the process and taught courses are as much about learning from one another as about the acquisition of facts. The loneliness that some people feel when doing an MD or PhD is not part of a taught course where one has peer support in abundance.

As well as varying in content the current courses vary in style. There are courses for GPs only, e.g. GKT, Birmingham and Keele, and multidisciplinary courses, e.g. Exeter, Sheffield, Nottingham, Queen Mary and Westfield College, University of London. Some are organised as *strands*, that is the students attend for a day a week in term time, and others as *modules*, that is the teaching takes place in blocks with additional home study in between. Most run over two to three years. There is now a distance-learning Masters, making extensive use of new technologies, run by the University of Derby. The University of Warwick runs a course on management in primary care, which is again multidisciplinary.

Since 1996 GPs taking taught Masters courses have been able to apply for a prolonged study leave grant from the Department of Health, provided they have the support of their director of postgraduate education for general practice, which is normally forthcoming. This is a once in a lifetime payment which covers locum costs for the duration of the course and writing up time. Most courses are approved for the Postgraduate Education Allowance for those who wish to use their prolonged study leave at another time, for example to pursue the research they have begun in their Masters course. For nurses employed by health authorities (e.g. district nurses and health visitors) sponsorship may be available from the employing authority. For practice nurses the position is a little more difficult as the amount paid by the health authority may not be commensurate with the nurse's salary, leaving the employing GPs to make up the shortfall, something which they may or may not be willing to do. Whoever is paying, the financial cost of the course is only part of the overall cost. There is time out from everyday work, which has to be made up by colleagues or by the individual at another time, time out in evenings and at weekends, there is the cost of travel, books and, sometimes, the research itself. All these factors need to be very carefully considered before embarking on such a course. As can be seen from the personal contributions to this chapter, joining a course, learning new things and meeting like-minded people can bring about change in the participants. Sometimes this can amount to a dissatisfaction with their working life and may cause some individuals to look at a change in career, at least for part of the time.

Graduates of taught courses go on to do all manner of things. For some the stimulation and change in their thinking is sufficient in itself and they return to primary care refreshed. For others this is the start of a new direction: in research, education or management. A taught Masters course is principally about personal and professional development in ways in which research higher degrees are not. For those looking for stimulation and change in a wide range of areas one of these courses can offer a huge amount.

MSc in General Practice, The University of Birmingham

Cathryn Thomas

In the late 1980s the West Midlands Regional General Practice Education Committee recognised a need within the region to provide experienced GP trainers with a course which would develop their potential personally and professionally and enable them to make an increased contribution to education and research within the region. Many GPs in their early forties had been training for some time and were looking for something to challenge their thinking and to learn new skills. This was also a time when, both within the region and nationally, it was recognised that there was a need for more research from primary care. The idea of a course for trainers evolved into a taught higher degree. By training GPs in research methods and what was then called 'clinical epidemiology', now more familiar as 'evidence-based medicine', the General Practice Education Committee believed that GPs would enhance postgraduate teaching within the region and teach and undertake research.

The first cohort of students started in October 1991. The course is open to GPs only. Initially we stipulated a period of five years in general practice as a requirement. However, we have found that for those who are intent on a career in academic general practice a taught course can be a good starting point and that length of experience is in fact not as essential as we first thought. The taught component of the course is run on Thursdays in term time: 30 weeks a year for two years. The three people who set up the course (Richard Hobbs, David Wall and John Wilmot) argued successfully with the university that there should be a third year available for students to write up their dissertation.

In common with most universities, Birmingham is encouraging modularisation of its courses. While this has obvious advantages, in that students can take one module at a time and may be able to transfer credits from other courses within the university and from other bodies, the most potent part of the learning experience of our course is meeting with other GPs over a two-year period and developing relationships and trust over that time. For GPs the way in which they can utilise study leave will vary from practice to practice. For some it is easier to be absent for a day a week, for others a block of two or three days is better. Therefore both strand and modular courses are probably needed.

AIMS OF THE COURSE

To enable students to understand the nature of research by:

- extending their knowledge of quantitative research methodologies and statistics
- extending their knowledge of qualitative research methodologies – as they are applied to problems and issues in epidemiology, sociology, psychology and other relevant disciplines
- enabling students to understand the role of research in the development and practice of good medicine.

To enable students to evaluate evidence, especially by:

- developing an understanding of principles and practice of evidence-based medicine
- developing skills, such as audit, which produce evidence for reflection
- facilitating students' understanding of evidence offered by patients during consultation and examination
- enabling students, especially in their written assignments, to draw together evidence from various sources, evaluate and present it.

To contextualise research from the wider world of medicine, especially by:

- developing an understanding of the relationship between the clinical problem and the psycho-social context in which it presents
- developing an understanding of how other disciplines, such as sociology, may be relevant to the medical practitioner.

To enable students to think logically and broadly about a range of problems using a variety of relevant disciplines, especially by introducing students to relevant types of knowledge and modes of enquiry beyond medicine such as in management, economics and general ethics.

To enable students to improve their understanding of teaching and learning, especially by:

- developing knowledge of good educational theory and practice
- developing knowledge of learning styles
- developing skills in presentation and small group participation
- developing skills in small group facilitation
- offering the opportunity for reflection and development.

The first principle of our course is that it should be fun. This is not to say that we do not expect a high degree of commitment and intellectual rigour from our students, we do. However, for busy doctors to take on an additional, time-consuming task which is expensive in direct and indirect ways, the course itself must be enjoyable as well as stimulating and challenging. Each day involves three one-and-a-half-hour teaching sessions which all contain some practical work by the students. We cover core subjects: critical appraisal and evidence-based medicine,

Table 9.1 Numbers of students by cohort and gender

	Male	Female
1991–3	16	2
1993–5	9	3
1995–7	6	8
1997–9	8	2

research methodologies, both quantitative (including epidemiology and statistics) and qualitative; sociology and psychology; health economics; management; learning and teaching; ethics; and clinical topics where there is controversy or debate. Within these areas each course is different as the students' interests and needs influence the content. Teachers are mainly drawn from the Department of General Practice at Birmingham but we draw on expertise throughout the university and colleagues from other institutions. We are anxious that our students are exposed to as many different disciplines as possible and encourage them to suggest speakers whom they would particularly like to hear. The only caveat to this is a prohibition on overseas flights!

We run a course every two years as we prefer to concentrate on one group of students at a time. One feature of the cohorts of students has been a relative paucity of female students (student numbers shown in Table 9.1). The reasons for this seem, at least in part, to have to do with the greater domestic responsibilities of women, but it also seems that women are less confident in their abilities to undertake a course such as this. Our experience is that there are, of course, no grounds for these anxieties.

We also include four residential modules for two days each. The first is at the start of the course and is concentrated on meeting as a group, the second is concerned with ethics and the third with teaching. For the fourth residential module the students are assessed on a presentation on any topic of their choice. This is one of six assessments students have to do. The university requires all Masters students to do a written examination, ours involves critical appraisal of a paper, data interpretation and designing a research proposal to solve a question. The other assessments are an audit, a literature review and an essay on a medical topic.

The students have to undertake a piece of original research and write this up as a dissertation. It has been interesting to see the changes in method towards qualitative techniques as the cohorts have gone through and these methods have gained acceptance and understanding in primary care. We have found that the writing up of the dissertation is something which students find difficult. Only two students (out of 44) have managed to complete within two years. The third year has proved essential and the support of colleagues during this time is a great spur to completion.

Students should emerge from a course such as this with a questioning attitude. They are much less likely to accept what they are told by specialist colleagues, health authorities or government. They want to appraise the evidence for themselves and come to their own conclusions. The course aims to teach them the skills to do this.

UMDS MSc in General Practice*

Nicky Britten and Graham Calvert

The origins of the UMDS MSc in General Practice reflect its location in a merged institution. In 1982 the medical schools of Guy's and St Thomas's hospitals had combined to form the United Medical and Dental School. The Professor of General Practice on the Guy's campus, Peter Higgins, was also the Regional Adviser for General Practice for the South Thames Regional Health Authority. Members of the Regional Adviser's team made a major contribution to the development and teaching of the MSc. On the St Thomas's campus the Professor of General Practice, David Morrell, had been involved with the running of the St Thomas's Fellowship scheme for local GPs.[1] Discussions about a possible MSc course based in the combined department began in the early 1980s. It was felt that the core subjects of such an MSc should not be the medical school disciplines which have traditionally dominated hospital medicine but rather those subjects, such as social science, which reflect the everyday work of GPs. In addition, it was felt important that a key component of the course should be research, both because critical reading and understanding of research papers was important and also because it was hoped that the MSc graduates would go on with their own research after the end of the course. The new course thus combined a long tradition of general practice research with considerable experience of postgraduate teaching of GPs and a broad philosophical approach to the discipline. Approval for the course curriculum was eventually gained from the Medical Faculty and the first students were admitted in October 1986.

The course is intended for practising general practitioners, and the entry requirements are a registerable medical qualification and eligibility for appointment as a principal in general practice. Given that the course aims to help GPs reflect on their work and develop their critical faculties, it is more suitable for experienced GPs than for those early in their careers. The exception to this rule is the young GP who has decided on an academic career, for which the MSc provides an academic training. The majority of MSc applicants are GPs with no previous experience of research who often express a lack of confidence in their own ability to complete an adequate research project.

The aims of the course are various. First, to help doctors develop a critical approach to practice by closely examining their own work, by learning about the work of others and by developing a critical approach to published work in order to improve their professional performance. Second, to increase students'

---

* Following the merger with King's College London, the course is now known as the GKT MSc in General Practice.

understanding of human learning by relating practice to various theories of learning. It is intended that such an understanding will help students with their own development and learning and with any teaching they may undertake. Third, the course also aims to increase students' understanding of human behaviour in relation to health and illness in order to gain greater insight into the behaviour and needs of their patients and healthcare professionals. Fourth, it is intended that students will develop skills necessary to enable them to identify the moral components of their work, the principles used to discuss these issues and their philosophical basis. Last but certainly not least, it is intended that the course will provide doctors with a training in research methods and with an appreciation of the existing body of research findings, in order to equip them to undertake their own research and critical enquiries. These aims loosely correspond with the five taught modules of the course: Principles and Practice; Process of Learning; Social Science; Medical Ethics; Epidemiology and Research Methods.

The course is taught by 11 tutors consisting of five general practitioners, three sociologists, two psychologists and one statistician. Thus although the students are all GPs, they are exposed to other perspectives as a result of the diverse backgrounds of the tutors. The social science teaching in particular opens up new intellectual horizons as well as introducing new methodologies. This in turn encourages students to consider a wide range of research questions and helps them to undertake research projects on topics they might not have previously considered. Examples of research projects clearly influenced by the social science module include a study of patients' somatic attributional styles and a study of health locus of control in general practice. Other studies with a less explicit influence include a study about encouraging patient participation in general practice consultations; a study about the ritual of the post-natal examination; and a study about general practitioners' reputations with their patients.

The teaching of research methods in particular has evolved since 1986. At first there was an emphasis on expert led presentations of large, well funded, multi centre studies carried out by experienced research teams over long periods of time. While these were important in conveying epidemiological concepts, they were unhelpful as role models for students' own research projects. The nature of the course has changed as a result of student feedback and there is now much more emphasis on research carried out in general practice and on hands-on experience. The course begins with two group projects in which the group formulates its own research questions, designs the data collection instruments, collects the data, carries out some analysis and writes the project up.[2] The first of these two group projects is based on quantitative methods and the second is based on qualitative methods. The intention is that, by the end of the second term, students should have hands-on experience of both quantitative and qualitative methods, in order to choose an appropriate methodology for their own research project. Teaching in the third term concentrates on evidence-based practice and the evaluation of research. In the last term topics to do with research funding, management and dissemination are covered. The course thus aims to prepare students for doing their own projects as well as helping them appraise the research carried out by others.

Protocols for students' own research projects are developed over the second and third terms. This process is started in group sessions during which ideas for projects are presented to the rest of the group and two tutors for discussion. During these sessions the tutors may make suggestions about relevant literature and possible supervisors. On the basis of each student's area of interest, they are matched with a tutor with whom they work on a one to one basis over the following year. For most students data collection begins at the end of the first year. The research projects reflect students' own experiences in general practice and give them an opportunity to investigate questions of practical relevance to their own work. Indeed, many research projects derive directly from actual problems encountered in practice. Examples include the views of cancer patients in relation to truth telling about their condition; what receptionists think and feel about their work; collaboration between community pharmacists and GPs; and the development of a patient-generated outcome measure for primary care. The projects use a diversity of methods, several using more than one. Most projects are based in students' own practices and are carried out with very little financial support. Some studies are supported by small grants to cover the cost of printing and postage of questionnaires, or the transcription of qualitative interviews. The main resources consumed are the supervision time and the protected time of the student.

Fifty per cent of the final assessment is given to the research project, and distinctions are awarded to those displaying exceptional quality. The other 50% is given to a written, case-based examination and a portfolio of written assignments completed over the first four terms. The aim of these assignments is to encourage students to make links between the academic content of the course and their everyday work. It is also aimed to rehearse the skills necessary for the completion of the research project. Thus for example, one of the assignments seeks to rehearse skills in literature searching, selection and analysis by asking students to review current evidence for hormone replacement therapy and to use this to formulate a practice policy. Statistical skills are rehearsed by asking students to analyse an existing database using a computer package. A further portfolio item seeks to encourage students to reflect upon the way research ideas evolve and develop by reference to subsequent drafts of their project protocol.

A follow up survey of MSc graduates carried out in 1996 enquired about continuing involvement with research and their subsequent careers.[3] Two-thirds of respondents reported that they were currently engaged in research. While only a fifth of students reported having published work relevant to general practice prior to starting the MSc, over a half reported having done so after completing the course. For some of these, publication was based on their MSc project. At the time of writing, there have been 33 articles published on the basis of MSc projects. A number of graduates have gone on to register for other degrees or diplomas including five who have registered for PhDs and seven for MDs. Following the MSc, two-thirds of respondents had some kind of academic commitment. Thus MSc graduates have made, and are continuing to make, a significant contribution to the research base of general practice.

M Med Sci in Primary Healthcare, Nottingham

Roland Petchey

In many respects, the origins and subsequent development of the Nottingham M Med Sci reflect (and frequently anticipate) some of the changes which general practice/primary care has undergone over the past decade. For instance, when reviewing the course planning documentation, one can detect traces of some of the debates about the identity of primary care and issues (some still not full resolved) which have characterised policy nationally.

In Nottingham, the idea of a taught masters course first surfaced – in writing, at least – late in 1986. This, of course, was the year that the policy spotlight began to play on primary care, with the publication of *Primary Care: an agenda for discussion.*[4] Nevertheless, it is clear that, initially at least, discussions about the course were motivated almost exclusively by concerns that were internal to general practice. Minutes of meetings were dominated by discussion of the educational needs of GPs, the advancement of general practice as an academic subject and the integration of academic and professional postgraduate education for GPs. These concerns were reflected by the course at this stage of planning: it was initially entitled 'M Sc in General Practice' and intended exclusively for general practitioners. However, within a month or two its provisional title had changed to 'Primary Care', and its intended audience had been expanded to include 'others involved in primary healthcare'. By January 1987, 'others' had been specified as 'general practice, dentistry, community nursing, medical social work and Family Practitioner Committee administration'. Subsequently, however, this commitment to multiprofessionalism appears to have wavered somewhat. A paper from March 1987 reverted to 'M Sc in General Practice' and GP exclusivity. Later that year, the doors to non-GPs were re-opened, but social workers and FPC administrators were missing from the list of eligible entrants. Nevertheless, by the time the course was eventually formally proposed in January 1988, the inclusion/exclusion debate had been resolved in favour of inclusion: not just graduates of medicine, dentistry and nursing, but also medical social work, pharmacy, teaching, healthcare planning and administration. The eventual title of the course reflected this commitment to multiprofessionalism – M Med Sci in Primary Healthcare.

Other features of the early prototypes, however, remained remarkably constant throughout this period and subsequently. Foremost was the emphasis on education and training in research methods but of equal importance was the commitment to the integration of theory and practice and to an interdisciplinary (as well as multiprofessional) approach. It has to be conceded, though, that (with the 20:20 vision of hindsight) early understandings of what constituted interdisciplinary education appear slightly restricted. An early draft of the syllabus was criticised

Table 9.2 M Med Sci entrants (1989–97) by profession and gender (%)

General practitioners	18 (35)
Community nurses	13 (25)
Physiotherapists and occupational therapists	10 (19)
Primary care managers	6 (12)
Other community professions	5 (10)
Total	52
Female	38 (73)
Male	14 (27)

for totally neglecting health economics, medical sociology, health education and health promotion (all were subsequently incorporated). Overall, however, the extent to which the planning process anticipated so many later developments in primary care is quite remarkable. This is indicated by the fact that subsequent revisions of the course have left its essential character almost entirely untouched. Its original aims and its objectives remain virtually unchanged, despite the transformation of primary care in the intervening period.

The first intake to the M Med Sci was in October 1989. Since then, there have been a further four cohorts. Given the small size of the Department of General Practice, it was felt that a biennial intake was appropriate, since it allows us to focus our resources on a single cohort of students at a time and to personalise their experience. Table 9.2 analyses the 52 entrants to date by profession and gender. It shows that although GPs have been the single largest professional group, they represent only one-third of the total intake. The next largest professional grouping consists of community nurses, followed by physiotherapists and occupational therapists. 'Other' professions have included community pharmacists, a dentist and an osteopath.

Overall, women have outnumbered men by almost three to one, which is probably a fair reflection of the gendered nature of the primary care workforce. There is only one exception to this trend: two-thirds of GPs have been male. This is surprising given the increasing recruitment of women into the general practice workforce during the 1980s, and the reasons for it are unclear. It may be a product of status differentials within partnerships, or it may reflect the additional child care responsibilities that young women GPs are likely to have. Be that as it may, the diversity of professional viewpoints that are represented in a typical intake is one of the distinctive features of the Nottingham M Med Sci. It is also regarded as a considerable strength, since it offers countless occasions for the development of understanding of alternative perspectives and the interchange of views during discussion of issues of current relevance to primary care. The view of many of the staff who have been associated with the course is that we simply provide structured opportunities for students to learn from each other. The resultant exposure of professional conventional wisdom to challenge from other viewpoints is routinely cited by students as one of the most stimulating aspects of their experience.

As it is presently constituted, the course is a two year part-time taught masters. Candidates must be graduates in medicine, dentistry, pharmacy, nursing, the biological sciences or social sciences. Although graduate status is the normal requirement, there is provision for non-graduate candidates (indeed, some of our most successful students have been non-graduates). Candidates must also be practising as a professional in primary healthcare. In keeping with its original mission, the course has one overall aim: to facilitate the development of the 'reflective practitioner' by equipping students with the skills and knowledge they require in order to reflect critically on their personal and professional practice, to analyse the contexts in which they function, and to initiate, manage and respond effectively to change.[5] This aim breaks down into three objectives:

1. to provide a structured introduction to theories and concepts drawn from a range of contributory disciplines relevant to primary healthcare
2. to stimulate critical and analytical reflection on professional practice
3. to develop skills in the collection, analysis and interpretation of primary care data.

While the bulk of the teaching of research methods is undertaken by staff located in the Department of General Practice, the course draws on academic expertise and professional experience distributed widely within and outside the university. The major disciplinary inputs come from economics, sociology, management, ethics and law, with others such as history and informatics also contributing. Other community-based services such as social work, psychiatry and healthcare of the elderly are incorporated as well into an exploration of roles, responsibilities and interfaces in community care. The course is taught by a range of methods but with the emphasis on student-centred learning. Within the framework of the specified curriculum, the flexibility and informality that characterise a small postgraduate course are routinely capitalised on to vary the curriculum content in response to student interests or a topic of current relevance.

The two taught research methods modules in the first year have a single aim: to develop students' understanding of the strengths and limitations of a wide range of research methodologies, both as critically informed *consumers* of published research and as research *practitioners* in their own right. These skills are developed in a variety of ways, including practical exercises and critical reading, but mainly through the design and execution of a piece of original research. During the first year students are allocated to a supervisor on the basis of a shared interest in a topic or a methodology, and they work with them, initially towards the development of a Research Proposal which is submitted at the end of the first year, and ultimately towards completion of the project at the end of the course. The Proposal consists of a review of the relevant literature, a clearly specified research question which has been logically derived from it, a reasoned choice of method for investigating the question and an outline timetable for the project. It is also expected that some preliminary work will have been done on designing questionnaires or other instruments. The bulk of the project is not expected to be executed until the second half of the second year, but early completion and formal assessment of the Proposal in this way has been found to be helpful (though not infallible!) in detecting serious design flaws, and identifying specific skills of data collection or analysis that require further development. Separating the conception and design of the research from its execution in this way also serves to signal to students the fundamental importance of the design phase in the research process.

Some idea of the range of student interests can be obtained from the following selection of recent thesis topics:

- Disembodiment, reembodiment and attachment: patient experience during recovery and therapy following stroke
- Does advice from a general practitioner increase safety equipment use and safety behaviour in families with children aged five and under? A randomised controlled trial
- Transition to adult services: the perspective of parents of children with physical or learning difficulties.

These titles also illustrate the diversity of methods and study designs, ranging from in depth interviews of physiotherapists and stroke patients, through to telephone interviews, home visits and postal surveys. A further feature of much of the research is its *applied* nature. Many students take advantage of the opportunity offered by the project to research a topic which is of practical relevance to themselves as primary care professionals, in addition to providing a methodological challenge and contributing to theoretical understanding of situations and processes encountered in primary care. Above all else, though, the research project is a learning exercise. The M Med Sci is a *taught* masters, not a masters by research. Mistakes (even fundamental ones) in design or execution are permitted, as long as there is awareness of them and evidence that the students concerned have learned from them. Even so, an encouraging number of dissertations have been found to merit further development, either towards a higher degree or publication.

As mentioned above, a core aim of the course is the development of the *reflective practitioner.* This means regarding the contributory disciplines (sociology, ethics, economics and the like) not simply as valid and coherent systems of knowledge in their own right, but as the source of insights which can be applied to professional practice, either as reflection-*on*-action (what Arendt terms a 'stop and think') or reflection-*in*-action.[6] Right from the outset, the integration of theory and professional practice had always been an aim of the M Med Sci, but only recently has the fact that it is occurring been explicitly recognised and formally assessed. In the (imaginatively titled) 'Reflection on Professional Practice' assessments students are asked, first, to identify some significant situation, event or interaction that they have encountered in the course of their professional practice. They are then required to identify relevant theories or concepts from one or more of the contributory disciplines and apply them to the analysis of the situation or interaction. Again, the sheer diversity of the student response is only hinted at by the following selection of topics:

- The ethics and economics of Health Authority resource allocation decisions
- Intra-partnership strains following the establishment of an out-of-hours GP co-operative
- The ethical implications of deregulation of an emergency contraceptive.

The aim throughout is, in Schon's words, 'to build bridges' between the two worlds of the university and professional practice in primary care to the enrichment of both.

Taught Masters courses

Adrian Freeman

It began with a picture in a GP comic. There was my old medical school with three or four earnest looking academics. The article below described a 'new Masters degree course in General Practice'. I had been in practice for three years. After the initial confusion, I felt that things were coming under control with my patients and partners and I was ready to look around for extra dimensions; GP training, golf, that sort of thing. I considered myself a normal, jobbing GP. I had no previous academic experience outside medical school and thought that research was for the clever doctors with brains much bigger than mine. I still had powerful memories from medical school. The cardiologist who felt that my incompetence with a stethoscope destined me to a career in orthopaedics and the professor of medicine who had had to seriously question whether I should ever be allowed to practise.

As I looked at the picture of the Alma Mater in the comic I recalled those happy memories and I thought, why not give it a go. Time had moved on and so had I. My practice was 180 miles from the old medical school. A few simple enquiries showed that, at that time, the only other Masters course exclusively for GPs was 200 miles away, so I put in the application for the old school thinking that I may be against strong opposition. I found out later that as this was the first intake, they were actually almost at the point of paying me to come. I wish they had, because a Masters degree is not cheap! For a simple start there are the course fees. At that time going to do a Masters was not an established activity and rounds and rounds of letters and searches of obscure charities for funds came up with nothing. The course fees are only a part of it though. There is the travel (if you don't live on the doorstep of the university), the books and a computer. You will also have to organise your time out of the practice. In real terms it is one day a week during the university terms, but add in the residential modules and other activities and it soon clocks up.

There were 18 of us on the course. There is no typical Masters degree student. We were a mix of ages, culture and sex and I was not the only one travelling from a long distance. Our practices were as diverse as we were. This was 'lesson one' of the course. Once you become a Principal, your contact with GPs from different localities, interests and practice types declines. As a rural GP you can sympathise with the single-handed inner city doctor, but when you are learning together you get a real insight and understanding of their situation and vice versa. A strong bonding in the group developed and we helped each other through individual difficulties.

What was the learning like? Well, our first piece of work was an essay. If you have been through an undergraduate and postgraduate course based on MCQs and short notes, when was the last time you wrote an essay? Never mind the content, our punctuation and grammar was appalling and we did not know it. I'm still not sure I do! Taking one step further back we learnt how to read. Using those lessons of critical reading, basic statistics and epidemiology, I am no longer flummoxed by the papers in our journals. Some are actually very interesting. The content of the course was wide and changed to meet our needs.

The course was examined and we would only receive the degree if we passed all the exams. Initially we became quite agitated. Tell us what we must learn, we cried. Learn what you want to, came the reply. Tell us what we should research, we cried. Find the answers to your own questions, came the reply. Slowly it dawned. This was adult, or postgraduate, learning. We all had curiosities, questions we wanted to answer. The course taught the method to answer those questions. The exams were to demonstrate that we knew how to answer questions, our questions, not theirs. I learned how to use a medical library properly. I was astonished to realise the pleasure I could have in following a trail of knowledge until I knew everything there was to know, but only with regard to my question. I had hit the limit of known information. To answer my question I had to do the research myself. With that realisation the chips I had on my shoulder from the humiliation of my undergraduate teaching began to slide away. The cardiologist and the professor of medicine knew nothing about my question. I was up there with them, actually ahead of them in some ways. Those giants who had haunted me shrank away.

That is the big message from a Masters course – liberation, confidence. Did it change me? Emphatically no say I. Definitely yes, say my wife, friends, partners, etc. Your personality does not change – so I am right. However, my outlook, way of working, curiosity and confidence has all changed – so they are right. I have no doubt that my patient care has improved, as have my management skills. The degree has been a stepping stone. I have gone on to continue research at the local university, fellowship by assessment, training, college examiner and many other things. The Masters degree gave me the self-awareness that I could do these things. The one thing that I regret is that it is over. Oh and I still don't know how to play golf.

UMDS MSc in General Practice: the student experience

Norma O'Flynn

The reasons for doing an MSc are probably as numerous and varied as the people who decide to do it. My undergraduate medical education was a traditional one – two and a half years of basic sciences, followed by over three years of clinical and allied subjects. I regretted that although I had spent longer at university than the average undergraduate, the education I received had not attempted to broaden my understanding of myself or the world I lived in. However, my trainee year and the preparation for the MRCGP exposed me to ideas of critical thinking, and to literature about how people behaved and to general practice literature. It seems strange to say I enjoyed preparing for an exam, but I did, and I knew that continued exposure to similar critical thought was necessary to enhance my professional life. Following my trainee year and some time doing locums, I started a post as a salaried principal in the practice which is the clinical base for the Department of General Practice at UMDS. For me the decision to do the MSc was a natural progression from the readings I had discovered as a trainee, combined with a post which allowed me protected time. I did not make enquiries about other courses – I knew the content of the MSc at UMDS was what I was looking for from talking to previous students and tutors, geographically I was on the spot and funding was available from regional funds.

The majority of participants were doing the course for their own growth and development – improvements in patient care were a secondary benefit. Reasons given included seeking a rekindling of interest in people and medicine, one practitioner wanted to attempt doing research in his own practice, but did not know how to start, others were considering or starting academic careers.

The most practical message from my experience is that the commitment required to complete the course should not be underestimated. There is an immense amount of reading for the seminars each week. The reading can be divided between the group, or one can choose to read only some of the readings recommended, but the seminars are of most benefit and interest if the time is spent discussing the material rather than summarising and explaining it to the other group members. Time is required to plan the seminars that are led by the students themselves and portfolio items also have to be written. Portfolio items were invariably written up during vacation time, as the deadlines for submission were at the start of the next term. Some students had protected time for study in addition to the time to attend the seminars, but I did not. I was always tired and all other aspects of my life took second place. Although I thoroughly enjoyed the course, I was glad when it came to an end as I could not have continued to work at the pace required.

What did I learn? In terms of everyday practice, I was introduced to literature from psychological and sociological worlds that give more insight into how patients (and doctors) behave than medical texts do. Studying the general practice literature puts the current issues in general practice into historical context and exposes the deficiencies in the evidence to support current practices. For those considering research, the skills practised are as valuable as the knowledge gained. I particularly valued the discipline of having to finish and submit a port-folio item by a given deadline, even when I knew it could be improved by a few extra hours work. Familiarity with library systems, literature searches and com-puters is an added bonus as most of my group had graduated long before computers became commonplace. The development of a personal research project with the support of a supervisor and the feedback of the group, encourages the practice of writing protocols, getting ethical approval and discovering what is and what is not possible. However the emphasis on the project in the final marking results in a need for the project to succeed, as well as being a learning experience.

There are a number of features of the UMDS course that deserve mention – it is not multidisciplinary; all the students are general practitioners; there is no choice in the modules studied; and the coursework is done in a closed group over the first four terms. The fact that we were all general practitioners was seen as a positive aspect by the members of my group. We shared a common educational experience, both at undergraduate and postgraduate levels, and now worked providing general medical care to patients in the community. In essence we came to the course as equals and felt safe enough with one another to allow free discussion and criticism of each other's views and practice. Between us we had experience of medical education in a number of countries, work experience in a variety of settings and types of practices. Although the emphasis on general practitioners could be attacked for being too narrow, our experience was that it allowed for detailed discussion and analysis of our work.

If I had had a choice in the modules I studied, I would have missed out on what for me was one of the best discoveries of the MSc – the module on the process of learning. It introduced me to a literature I would never have known existed, let alone encountered. The module not only discussed what self-directed learning was about but put the principles into action, resulting in much awkward feeling as students realised what taking responsibility for one's learning really meant. This is not an argument for no choice for students in the modules they study, but a suggestion that exposure to subjects not previously considered can be interesting and worthwhile.

The UMDS MSc is based almost entirely on group work. The success and content of the sessions is dependent on the cohesiveness of the group and this is fostered by its closed nature. At its best the group worked autonomously and the realisation that we could critically analyse the literature using our own experience as general practitioners was a powerful step in demystifying research. The group was central to my enjoyment and learning and the support received from others who were similarly balancing practice and personal lives was immense.

It isn't necessary to do an MSc to explore the literature or learn the skills mentioned, but I found the direction and support provided by tutors invaluable.

The impetus of both the course and the other students pushes you to read further and to challenge your own perspectives.

References

1. Courtenay MJ, Morrell DC and Watkins CJ (1982) Fellowships in general practice in St Thomas's district. *BMJ.* **284**: 318–20.

2. Ogden J, Andrade J, Eisner M *et al.* (1997) To treat? To befriend? To prevent? Patients' and GPs' views of the doctor's role. *Scandanavian Journal of Primary Health Care.* **15**: 114–17.

3. Calvert G and Britten N (1998) The UMDS MSc in General Practice: attainment of intended outcomes. *British Journal of General Practice.* **48**: 1765–8.

4. Secretary of State for Health and Social Services (1986) *Primary Care: an agenda for discussion.* HMSO, London.

5. Schon DA (1987) *Educating The Reflective Practitioner.* Jossey-Bass, San Francisco.

6. Arendt H (1971) *The Life of The Mind. Vol 1: Thinking.* Harcourt Brace Jovanovich, San Diego.

10

RCGP Scientific
Foundation Board

Ross Taylor, Fenny Green and Bonnie Sibbald

BACKGROUND

The Royal College of General Practitioners' Scientific Foundation Board was established in 1976 and has charitable status. The Board's capital comes from two major sources. These are the General Fund, which was created following a major appeal in 1980 for funds to support all types of general practice research, and a number of Special Funds, which support research in specific areas and which are mostly funded from legacies. The largest of these special funds is the Windebank Fund for diabetes-related research.

The annual amount available for distribution by the Board is the interest obtained from the investment of its capital funds. The level of the Board's income can, therefore, fluctuate but it is generally somewhere in the region of £60 000 to £70 000 a year from its General Fund and about £30 000 from its Special Funds. As its income fluctuates, the Board has from time to time to review the maximum amount which it will normally award. For example, it decided in 1996 to raise this sum to £10 000 from the £5000 it had been since 1974. (Up to £30 000 may, however, be available for diabetes-related research only (Windebank Fund).)

MEMBERSHIP

The Board's members are appointed by the Council of the RCGP and the majority are members of the College. Some are appointed from outside the College's membership, in particular those with a special expertise in statistics and the social sciences. All members of the Board are experienced researchers. Professor John Howie has recently succeeded Professor David Morrell as Chairman.

POLICY

The Board awards grants for research which is of direct relevance to general practice and which is undertaken within the UK. Priority is given to short-term projects, which will normally last up to 18 months, and to pilot projects.

Increasingly, the major funding bodies (research councils, major charities and NHS R&D) direct their funds towards research in predetermined priority areas. It is worth noting that the SFB has no research priorities of its own and is therefore one of the few remaining sources of funding for interesting ideas which are outside of the current 'directed research' agenda.

The Board recognises that it is often difficult for new or relatively inexperienced researchers to obtain funding from other sources where they are having to compete against well established researchers. It therefore gives high priority to applications from young and/or new researchers and to those who have not previously been funded by the Board. There is a corresponding expectation that those who have been 'given a start' by the Board will move on to obtain future funding from other sources, so that repeated applications are likely to meet with decreasing success and encouragement to apply elsewhere.

The Board will consider applications from any discipline for funding for projects which are directly relevant to general practice/primary care, but it does give high priority to submissions from practising general practitioners and other members of the primary healthcare team.

ROLE OF THE BOARD

The Board is not only a grant awarding body. It has an important role in advising and guiding researchers. The Board works closely with the College's National Research Adviser (currently Professor Paul Freeling), who attends its meetings as an observer. He is available, by arrangement with the Clerk to the Board, to comment on research proposals and applications to the Board prior to their submission. The National Research Adviser receives copies of all the applications received for funding but does not have a vote when awards are being decided.

THE ASSESSMENT PROCESS

The Board meets three times a year in January, May and October. Submissions for grants in excess of £1000 are assessed by all members of the Board. Reports are submitted and collated well in advance of each meeting at which an agreed view is reached on each submission. A separate fast-track process for applications for less than £1000 uses the same application form but awards are made at the discretion of the Chairman or, in his absence, the Honorary Secretary.

Members of the Board examine the personal information provided by the applicant (including a brief curriculum vitae) to assess the amount of research experience he or she has and the support facilities to which they will have access while doing their project. Members consider whether the aims of the project or the proposed research question are clearly stated; they consider the value of the proposed project with regard to what it will add to the body of scientific knowledge; and examine the proposed methods, looking particularly to see whether they are appropriate and whether the applicant is aware of any inherent problems which may be associated with his or her selected approach.

Inexperience is not a disadvantage, provided that applicants show that they have a good chance of success, through willingness to seek advice and to arrange suitable support.

THE OUTCOMES OF THE ASSESSMENT PROCESS

The assessment process leads to a number of possible outcomes. These are: unconditional funding with no reservations, unconditional funding with comments/ suggestions, funding subject to certain conditions, moderate amendments, interview, resubmission and rejection. There is a wide range of reasons why candidates may be asked to attend for interview but the general purpose is to allow the candidate the opportunity to clarify any issues which might otherwise preclude award of funding. The assessment process is not just a decision-making process about whether or not a project should receive funding. It is a valuable means of providing advice and guidance to applicants and this is reflected in the number of possible outcomes.

Increasingly, many applications are of a high standard and the Board funds these unconditionally. The Board does, however, encourage and receive applications from new or relatively inexperienced researchers and this may be reflected in the content of their application. In such cases the Board will reply to the applicant saying why they are not in a position to support the application in its current form, for example indicating the areas of the research protocol which need to be reviewed or highlighting aspects on which the applicant needs to obtain further advice.

In 1996 the Board received 48 applications of which 36 (75%) were funded (Table 10.1). Box 10.1 gives extracts from letters to applicants from the Honorary Secretary to illustrate the type of comment and advice which may be given by the Board.

The Board's intention is to provide constructive criticism and helpful advice to applicants to enable them to write a well thought out and good-quality research

Table 10.1   Grants awarded in 1996

Name and Study	Award
Dr R Gadsby Aetiology of pregnancy sickness and symptom complex – a pilot study for a new methodological approach for investigating the aetiology	£4339.00
Ms MA Durand and Dr MB King Interventions for women with abnormal attitudes to eating – a randomised controlled trial	£5182.00
Dr T Fahey Systematic review and meta-analysis of the treatment of acute bronchitis in general practice Systematic review and meta-analysis of the treatment of seborrhoeic dermatitis with imidazole antifungal agents	£4383.44
Dr Ruth Pinder and Dr David Lloyd Part-time women in general practice: from experience to participation in shaping professional development	£5000.00
Dr Tim Coleman A comparison of general practice consultations which are video-recorded with those which are not: patient characteristics and clinical content	£999.97
Dr Elizabeth Muir A study of the attitudes and behaviour of vocational trainees and their trainers towards persons with congenital disabilities by questionnaire and critical incident interview	£995.00
Dr Jane Ogden Predicting dietary regulation in patients with non-insulin dependent diabetes mellitus following a consultation with a primary healthcare professional WINDEBANK FUND	£27 205.00
Dr Jim Cox Randomised placebo controlled trial of oral salbutamol for nocturnal cough in children: pilot study	£9659.29
Dr A Farmer The impact of screening for non-insulin dependent diabetes mellitus on psychological wellbeing and attitude to health WINDEBANK FUND	£26 211.00
Dr L Mountford Crime and health – patients' perceptions of the link	£630.00
Dr SD Smith General practitioners' perceptions of their information needs and problems involved in teaching basic clinical skills to undergraduate medical students within a community setting	£693.00

Table 10.1 Continued

Name and Study	Award
Dr N Oswald The clinical review of atrial fibrillation: what are the consequences of an attempt to get research into practice (GRIP)?	£3726.00
Dr C Paterson MYMOP as a patient-held record: experience and views of patients and practitioners	£1987.00
Dr M Aylett What advice and support on research is available to primary healthcare teams?	£3232.00
Dr S de Lusignan and Dr S Quick Pilot study to establish guidelines for the management of urinary symptoms in males over 50 in primary care	£1000.00
Dr S Grieve Violent incidents in general practice and primary care	£4968.00
Dr PF Bleiker What do general practitioners think of extending the role of community pharmacists?	£630.00
Dr N Beale Drawing the flak – primary healthcare team members acting as customer relations officers for the NHS	£2013.00
Dr J Spitzer in collaboration with Dr L Neville Group A streptococcal carriage in North Hackney with particular reference to the Orthodox Jewish Community	£6319.20
Dr J Cornwell A qualitative study to explore general practitioners' knowledge and attitudes to the treatment of depression	£2000.00
Dr UT Kadam Mental health needs in a practice population: an epidemiological survey of needs and health care services utilisation, and a qualitative investigation of patients' views of health needs	£5000.00
Dr C Cornford How patients on long-term oxygen treatment cope with their illness: a qualitative study	£2287.00
Dr M Gray The acceptability of screening sigmoidoscopy	£3550.00
Dr M Jones An RCT of CME on management of acute myocardial infarction for GP deputies	£1200.00
Dr R Gregg Academic general practitioners and practice development in deprived areas	£957.00

Table 10.1   Continued

Name and Study	Award
Dr J Chen The primary care pharmacist as the patient's drug adviser: a useful addition to the primary healthcare team?	£984.25
Dr EM Saunderson The beliefs, role and expectations of general practitioners to the recently bereaved: idiosyncrasy or planned intervention?	£1000.00
Dr S Saxena A survey of the prevalence of contraceptive use, knowledge of contraceptive techniques and attitudes to their use in Asian women in two general practices in south London	£1607.50
Dr C Butler A case study of nurse management of acute illness: impact on help-seeking behaviour with upper respiratory tract infections	£5000.00
Dr JL Campbell Inherited defective colour vision and clinical care – does colour blindness make a difference?	£3250.00
Dr N Landi Health beliefs, attitudes and knowledge of diabetes mellitus in Gujeratis	£2239.25
Dr H Weinbren Health beliefs and attitudes in families of children with epilepsy	£1839.25
Dr A Gilliland, Dr K Steele and Dr JS Brown A retrospective study to gather information about patients removed and assigned to general practitioners in Northern Ireland over a 12-year period (1985–96)	£3404.76
Dr J Thistlethwaite Community-based teaching of undergraduate medical students: what effect does it have?	£4982.00
Dr J Thistlethwaite The triple test: understanding and experience in one general practice	£4792.54
Dr N O'Flynn Menorrhagia in general practice: the patient's perspective	£975.00

protocol and application for funding. The ability to write a high-quality application is an essential prerequisite if researchers are to go on to be successful in obtaining funds from other grant awarding bodies in strong competition with experienced research workers.

Box 10.1   Examples of comments and advice

(a) Unconditional funding with suggestions from the Board

'… I am pleased to inform you that the Board generally agreed that you had prepared an extremely good application and unanimously agreed to award funding for your project. The only point the Board would like me to make is that in drawing conclusions from your work you will need to take account of the fact that only one nurse is involved and her personal qualities and skills, including her already established relationship with patients, will be a major variable in themselves. There will be difficulty in separating the effect of nursing skills in general from the personal qualities of this particular nurse. There might, therefore, be a need for a subsequent, much larger study, in order to confirm that your findings have external validity (i.e. can be extrapolated to other settings). We are, however, happy to fund this as a very well designed pilot study and award you a sum up to a maximum of £5000 in respect of the secretarial, postage, printing and stationery, and telephone costs.'

(b) Funding subject to conditions

'… I am pleased to inform you that the Board is prepared to support your project but I have been asked to obtain some additional information and assurances before funding is actually granted. Members of the Board were concerned that this was a particularly delicate and sensitive area which would require particular care and sensitivity on the part of an interviewer. We would like to be assured that you will have the support and supervision of a senior qualitative researcher who has considerable experience of interviewing techniques in these sensitive areas. I would therefore be grateful if you could identify a suitable supervisor and ask him or her to write to us with an undertaking to that effect. We would then be prepared to release the funds which have been voted in principle.'

NOTIFICATION OF FUNDING DECISIONS

The Board's decision will normally be notified to the applicant within two weeks of the relevant meeting. Requests for up to £1000 can be considered at any time during the year under the Chairman's action process. Applicants will normally receive a decision from the Chairman within four weeks of the application being received. This system enables applicants seeking small grants, perhaps for a pilot project or to fund a research project undertaken as part of a Masters degree, to receive a rapid response.

ADVICE FOR APPLICANTS

The Board supplies a set of guidelines to applicants to assist them in completing their application form. This covers issues such as eligibility, the size of grant available, the type of expenditure which the Board is prepared to fund and guidance on the level of detail to be included in the application. With the new or relatively inexperienced researcher particularly in mind, the guidelines contain a section which highlights some of the common reasons why the Board will either reject or require amendment to an application.

Although the Board explicitly recognises the special difficulties that general practitioners may have in establishing themselves as researchers, it is nonetheless accountable for the efficient expenditure of its limited resources. Board members will look in particular for evidence of 'value for money', i.e. that a useful outcome will be achieved, compatible with the amount of funding awarded. The highest levels of outcome would be definitive results that could influence the practice of primary care, but other lesser levels of outcome are often more appropriate. These particularly include 'pump priming' for an eventual major study. Applicants are advised to be explicit about the aims of this kind of preparatory work. A major literature review might be necessary to clarify the questions to be asked. A systematic review of previous work could be funded if it had not already been done. Preliminary studies might be needed to test the feasibility of methods, e.g. identifying and contacting appropriate patients, acceptability of questionnaires, etc. Wherever possible, existing instruments should be used because the development and validation of new questionnaires is beyond the scope of this level of application (although our practical experience section includes a notable exception). The next stage – a pilot study – is generally considered to be a 'dry run' on a small scale, to assess response rates and other possible operational problems (exemplified by Chris Butler's account in the practical experience section). Many of the projects which SFB funds are at this 'pilot' level. The final step from pilot to main study is often a large one. The population of a single practice is rarely adequate and specialist advice (especially on sampling and sample size) is essential.

Some of the commoner problems with applications are summarised in Box 10.2.

Lastly, the amounts or kinds of funding requested may be considered inappropriate. Applications should generally be within the current limits for total funding. Apart from that, the Board cannot, for example, fund locum expenses. It also does not usually fund research training (for which there are other sources of funding) and it cannot reimburse, in full, expenses for attendance at conferences. It is, however, prepared to meet 50% of conference fees and related expenses for events within the UK up to a maximum of £250. Applications for special equipment (computers, dictaphones, etc.) need to be carefully justified and, where applicants are supported by universities or other institutions, we might expect such equipment to be already available. These conditions may be changed from time to time to reflect changes in the Board's policy or other external factors. Because of its

---

Box 10.2   Problems with applications

- *Insufficient detail:* some applications may put up a good idea but simply give so little detail of background and method that Members cannot judge its quality
- *Insufficiently aware of previous work:* you should show that you know of major previous work and a concise literature review should identify the main issues and the 'gap' that your proposed study will fill
- *Aims unclear:* there need not be a hypothesis as such, but there should be a well-stated purpose. Members look for a clear research question which they will then try to match with your 'Methods' section to assess how likely you are to be able to answer the question
- *Faults in method:* the whole design may be at fault but more commonly it is some aspect of methods, with sampling coming top of the list. A good source of advice on sampling methods and (if appropriate) sample size and power calculations is needed for many studies

---

charitable status, the SFB does not fund central institutional overheads, e.g. university on-costs for central services and/or administration.

FINAL REPORTS

As a condition of their award, everyone who is awarded a grant is required to submit a short report within 12 months of the expected end date of their project. The report consists of a structured abstract of around 500 words describing the project; a list of project outputs including oral and written presentations; an indication of whether the project formed part of research toward a higher degree; and a brief explanation of any departures from the anticipated budget or timetable. All project reports are read by a member of the Board who may occasionally write to grant-holders offering critical feedback or seeking additional information. Information on the outcome of previous projects is taken into account in considering subsequent applications from the same person.

Project reports are abstracted into a computer database which is used to produce a performance report presented annually to the Board. These annual performance reports serve a number of useful purposes. They enable the Board to assess the value of Scientific Foundation Board awards in terms of generating high-quality research publications, enabling novice researchers to attain higher degrees, and disseminating research through meetings and lectures to a wider audience of primary healthcare professionals. Reports for the period 1990–5, for example, indicate that about two-thirds of projects were disseminated at meetings and conferences, half were published in leading scientific journals and a third contributed to higher degrees. Any changes in performance can be identified and problems rectified, where appropriate, by modifying the guidance to applicants or awards procedures. For example, the Board clarified its budget planning advice to applicants after performance reports suggested that grant-holders were getting into financial difficulty through failing to anticipate salary rises for project employed staff. Finally, the performance reports are useful in demonstrating the value of the Scientific Foundation Board to the College and to potential donors. Only by sustaining a good record of performance can the Board expect to merit continued and growing support.

Practical experience

Chris Butler

The first research grant I won was from the Scientific Foundation Board of the RCGP and I see it as a major milestone in my efforts to develop a career in academic general practice. Winning this grant to develop a brief counselling intervention against smoking for use in general practice helped me win a larger grant for a randomised clinical trial. The experience of having written one grant application was invaluable when it came to constructing the application for the larger grant. The fact that I had already won money for development work from a prestigious scientific body probably impressed the committee who awarded the larger grant. This larger study is forming the basis of an MD thesis.

I won a second grant from the SFB to explore the impact of nurse intervention on help-seeking behaviour for upper respiratory tract infections. I knew of a nurse who had just been appointed in a nearby practice to see acute, minor cases and I was keen to make use of this opportunity for a natural experiment. I wanted money fairly quickly to do a study of feasibility: I knew that a study on this scale would by no means be the final answer to the question of efficacy. I also wanted to get experience of the nuts and bolts of researching this area (e.g. what problems might there be in obtaining the relevant data from clinical records?) and to develop and pilot appropriate questionnaires and measures for assessing outcomes.

Formal randomisation of patients was not feasible in this practice, given limited research resources. The SFB could see beyond the obvious imperfections of this small preliminary study and did not get fixated on the imperfect (but non-disruptive to the practice) procedure for allocation of patients. I now have experience and data from over 400 patients which will greatly strengthen any future application for a larger grant to evaluate similar interventions using more traditional research methods.

Writing a proposal for a small grant involves the same processes as for a bigger grant: the sum might be different, but the rationale, study design, timetabling and budgeting have to be just as rigorous.

The SFB has given a kick-start to many researchers and research programmes in British general practice. More than any other grant-giving body, this Board is likely to understand the complexities and unique problems that researchers face when doing general practice-based research. I have found them approachable and sympathetic and their feedback has improved my study protocols. They have also suggested individuals who are prepared to help with particular problems in study design (e.g. statisticians). The SFB is the ideal first port of call for the young practitioner to launch a research career, or for those who wish to obtain support for pilot and small projects which have a typical general practice flavour that other grant-giving bodies are unlikely to appreciate in full.

Charlotte Paterson

I was a general practitioner with 18 years of practice experience but no academic training who was starting out on clinical research. I needed all the help I could get. The research ideas came from my primary healthcare team, who have remained throughout a bedrock of support and enthusiasm.

A Master's degree course at the Department of General Practice, UMDS (London), provided me with a grounding in research skills, and my tutors there helped me to formulate a detailed protocol for my project. This was to design and start validation of a new patient-generated outcome measure for primary care, called 'Measure Yourself Medical Outcome Profile' (MYMOP).

My first funding application for this project was rejected and the funding body in question told me that as I was a GP with no research experience I was unlikely to succeed, and advised me to work in collaboration with experts in health measurement. I learned two lessons from this rebuff. First, that seeking funding was more than seeking money; it was also to do with seeking a vote of approval from my profession. Second, that within the medical research establishment, GPs were still struggling for their voices to be heard. It was with these thoughts in mind that, in the summer of 1994, I turned to the Royal College of General Practitioners and applied to the Scientific Foundation Board for a grant of just over £1000. When this application was successful, and was backed by a bursary of £500 from the Royal Society of Medicine, not only was I relieved that my project could now go ahead on a proper footing and with some secretarial support, but I felt strengthened for the task ahead.

The successful completion of this project, and the resulting dissertation and paper in the *BMJ*[1] have laid a solid foundation for our practice research programme.[1] We have been successful in our application to become a South and West Region research general practice, MYMOP questionnaires and support have been sent out to more than 50 researchers and I am currently extending my research training towards a doctorate. This time, when we needed funding, I knew immediately where to go, and our present project, which is investigating both the practicality of presenting MYMOP in a patient-held record and the patients' views on its use, is being funded by a second grant of nearly £2000 from the SFB. My relief and pleasure at receiving this second grant was just as great as before and, although I now appreciate that these sums are considered small grants, my experience is that they make all the difference between sinking and floating. They provide a helping hand on the most difficult steps of all: those first ones.

REFERENCE

1. Paterson C (1996) Measuring outcomes in primary care: a patient-generated measure, MYMOP, compared with the SF-36 health survey. *BMJ.* **312**: 1016–20.

11

Association of University Departments of General Practice

John Campbell and Alison Wilson

*'Excellence in Teaching and Research in
General Practice and Primary Care'*

Although there are now 38 departments of general practice/primary care throughout the UK, the discipline represents one of the youngest university medical specialties with responsibility for both teaching and research. It was not until 1953 that the first independent university department of general practice was created in Edinburgh. Since that time, there has been considerable development within each of the 25 UK medical schools with responsibility for undergraduate medical education and among an increasing number of those institutions which have involvement in postgraduate medical education. Academic challenges presented in the fields of primary care teaching and research are the subject of enthusiastic and innovative investigation within these departments. The Association of University Departments of General Practice (AUDGP) is a thriving coalition of medical and non-medical colleagues from a wide variety of disciplines; all have an interest in the delivery of primary care to the population. Recent years have seen an encouraging growth in the breadth and depth of the activities of the Association which represents the interests of the wider disciplines of academic general practice and primary care. Patients as well as undergraduate and postgraduate students benefit from the ongoing and increasing expertise of colleagues based in university departments of general practice and primary care.

Primary Care

Primary care is defined as the provision of integrated, accessible healthcare services by clinicians who are accountable for addressing a large majority of personal healthcare needs, developing a sustained partnership with patients and practising in the context of a family and a community. In the UK most first-contact healthcare occurs in general practice; on average there are about four contacts per patient per year with a general practitioner; 90% of medical care in the UK is provided by GPs. Primary care is also provided by practice nurses, nurse practitioners, health visitors and district nurses, midwives, optometrists, dental practitioners and a range of other professions allied to medicine.

Primary care is important because it functions between self-care of common problems in the community, and the use of expensive secondary and tertiary (hospital) resources. There is good evidence that cost-effective healthcare systems are characterised by a strong primary care sector in which GPs and family physicians exercise a gatekeeping role, judiciously controlling access to hospital services and providing diagnostic and therapeutic interventions at an appropriate technological level in primary care.

The Secretary of State for Health in the UK has emphasised the importance of a 'primary care-led NHS' in which the needs of patients in communities, identified by GPs and others working in primary care settings, will be used as a basis for the commissioning of primary, secondary and tertiary care services. This health needs assessment process takes place in the context of major changes in the structure of the UK NHS with the introduction in the early 1990s of a split in the purchaser and provider functions of organisations within the NHS. Alternative models for commissioning care are presently under investigation. If the commissioning process is to be clinically appropriate and cost-effective, it must be informed by research-based information and clinical effectiveness, emphasising the need for a vigorous academic base to support clinical general practice.

The late 1990s have seen the focus of clinical care move from the hospital to general practice, and this 'secondary:primary care shift' has major implications for skills, resources and professional roles within primary care. Investigations and treatments which, until only a few years ago, were the exclusive province of the hospital specialist, are now routinely undertaken in general practice; hospital stays are becoming shorter and more postoperative and postdischarge care is required in the community. As the clinical focus shifts from hospital to primary care, so the academic focus follows, and there have been calls from many bodies to ensure that medical students in training are given extended teaching and learning opportunities in primary care. Significant proportions of the total undergraduate curriculum in many medical schools are now pursued in general practice and primary care settings. On a similar vein, there is an increasing need to focus research around primary care and to develop the skills of primary care researchers.

ACADEMIC GENERAL PRACTICE AND THE AUDGP

The first Chair of General Practice in the UK was founded in 1963 and taken up by Professor Richard Scott in Edinburgh. Since that time almost every medical school in the UK has established a department of general practice, sometimes free-standing, sometimes derived from and related to a department of community health or public health medicine, but always with a clear focus on providing teaching for undergraduates in the setting of general practice and the pursuit of research in general practice involving multidisciplinary teams.

A 'typical' department of general practice will consist of a core group of academic staff, led by a professor and a number of senior lecturers, supported by lecturers in general practice, and including teaching and research staff drawn from other disciplines, such as nursing, health psychology, medical sociology, bio-statistics, anthropology and from the other life and social sciences. The non-medical membership of departments of general practice and primary care reflects the multidisciplinary nature of general practice itself and the commitment to the development of multiprofessional work. Most departments in the UK are practice-linked, that is to say the core department is situated in the medical school, with clinical academics undertaking their general practice duties in a number of linked practices some distance from the university. Five departments (Edinburgh, Manchester, Southampton, Cardiff and UMDS, London) are practice-based; these practices are staffed by a group of GPs who all hold academic appointments in the department of general practice, and the research and teaching facilities are incorporated into the same building as the practice.

Hitherto, entry to academic general practice for general practitioners has generally been at lecturer level following a period of vocational training and practice-based experience. There are however increasing numbers of examples of schemes providing extended vocational training for general practitioner registrars. Several of these schemes involve placement in, or association with an academic department of general practice/primary care.[1] Such arrangements provide opportunities for recently trained practitioners who wish to develop research and teaching skills prior to becoming a principal GP or securing an academic appointment.

The AUDGP has proposed a career structure for academic general practice and is contributing to discussions on a parallel structure for GPs involved in postgraduate education. Lecturers may expect to spend around five years learning about teaching methods and undertaking original research towards a higher degree, while undertaking clinical general practice work for about 50–60% of their time, before applying for a senior lectureship. At this level, comparable to a consultant in NHS clinical practice, most clinical academic GPs will possess a higher degree, have experience in undertaking research and obtaining significant research grants, will probably have developed a special research interest, will have expertise in teaching and will be spending 30–40% of their time in direct clinical patient care. Progression to a Chair usually requires about 5–7 years of experience as a senior lecturer. Professors of general practice are likely to spend the majority of

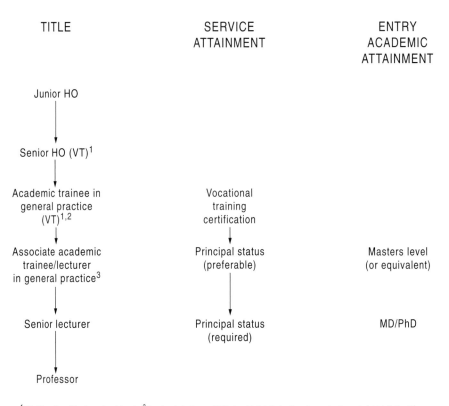

TITLE	SERVICE ATTAINMENT	ENTRY ACADEMIC ATTAINMENT
Junior HO		
Senior HO (VT)[1]		
Academic trainee in general practice (VT)[1,2]	Vocational training certification	
Associate academic trainee/lecturer in general practice[3]	Principal status (preferable)	Masters level (or equivalent)
Senior lecturer	Principal status (required)	MD/PhD
Professor		

[1]VT=Vocational trainee (registrar). [2]Academic trainees (VT) should distribute time in each of years 4 and 5 equally between clinical and academic duties. [3]This would be the general practice equivalent of a senior (specialist) registrar in hospital practice. In many cases lecturers will have partner and principal status.

Figure 11.1 Proposed core academic career structure (after Fraser *et al.*[2])

their time in a leadership capacity and are expected to undertake national and international academic work. Typically, they continue to spend 20–30% of their time in patient care.

Many non-medical members of departments of general practice and primary care come into the field with degrees and/or relevant experience in health service work. Their career structure follows one of two possible routes. As research associates or research fellows, their career pathway may lead to promotion to senior research associate or professor of primary care research following a number of years of primary care research experience and attainment of substantial research grants and publications. Alternatively, others who play a leading role in teaching as well as research are employed as lecturers and may progress to a Chair following a number of years experience in organising and delivering teaching for medical undergraduates as well as developing their own research programmes.

Unlike the general practitioner department members, non-medical staff rarely have clinical responsibilities, although a recent survey of nurses in academic departments of general practice and primary care, supported by the AUDGP, highlighted the need to provide clinical opportunities for nursing staff. The AUDGP has an active non-medical group and is reviewing the career progression of this growing group of members. In the context of the primary care-led NHS and the NHS Research and Development programme, it is essential that inter-professional working at academic and practice levels is developed. Academic departments of general practice and primary care in the late 1990s have established broad-based multiprofessional teams which will enable the medical challenges of the future to be met.

Growth

The AUDGP is the professional association of members of academic departments of general practice, or their equivalent, in the UK and Republic of Ireland. Membership of the Association is open to all full-time and part-time academic staff of university departments of general practice, whether medically qualified or not. The Association was first formally constituted in 1974 when it had a membership of less than 50; in 1996 the membership was 540, distributed amongst 37 departments of general practice/primary care. The expansion and development of the Association is a reflection of the rapid growth which has taken place within academic general practice in the last 25 years.

In 1972, only 11 of the 29 UK medical schools had an academic general practice presence, and there were only six professors of general practice. Dr Robert Harvard Davis (Cardiff) initiated and convened a meeting in his department which led to the establishment of the Association of University Teachers in General Practice, the forerunner of the present Association. The first scientific meeting of the Association was held in Manchester in 1973, when Professor Pat Byrne became the first chairman of the newly formed Association with John Howie the first secretary. A formal constitution was agreed in 1974.

Considerable expansion in personnel and broadening of the activities of departments of general practice has underpinned recent developments. By 1996, all 32 UK undergraduate medical schools had academic departments of general practice or the equivalent, and there were 30 professors of general practice.

The composition of the membership of departments of general practice, and of the Association has altered dramatically over the years. Initially, every member was medically qualified in contrast with the present day when 25% of the membership is drawn from social and behavioural scientists and members of the professions allied to medicine. The most recent category of membership comes from the postgraduate departments of general practice in universities which do not have responsibility for the undergraduate education of medical students.

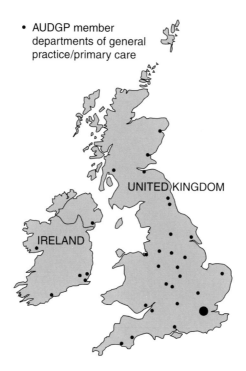

- AUDGP member departments of general practice/primary care

UNITED KINGDOM

IRELAND

Figure 11.2 Distribution of 38 departments of general practice/primary care in the UK and Ireland

STRUCTURE

The membership of the Association delegates the day-to-day activities to an executive body with three recognised officers: Chairman, Secretary and Treasurer. In addition to the three officers, the Executive comprises seven elected members of the Association and a further four non-elected members of the Executive representing the heads of departments, the Royal College of General Practitioners, the UK Postgraduate Advisers in General Practice and the department hosting the forthcoming scientific meeting. Further members may be co-opted at the discretion of the Executive. The Association is represented on the Council of the Royal College of General Practitioners and the Joint Committee on Postgraduate Training in General Practice, and at the United Kingdom Conference of Postgraduate Advisers in General Practice. Advice and expert opinion is provided regularly to strategic planning groups at the UK Department of Health.

While membership of the Association is open to a wide range of personnel from departments of general practice, the Heads of Departments' Group is an informally constituted body, closely linked with the Association, and representing all heads of departments of general practice/primary care. This group meets twice a year for discussion of matters relating to overall strategy, financing and development of the discipline within the UK university structures.

CONSTITUTION

A formal constitution was agreed in 1974, and has been modified on numerous occasions since that time at the Annual General Meeting of the Association. The constituency of the Association consists of members of university departments (or their equivalent) whose aims are in accordance with those of the Association. Distinction is drawn in the constitution between those departments who have responsibility for a programme of undergraduate medical student education, as compared with those without this responsibility.

Box 11.1   Aims of the AUDGP (1996)

- To promote teaching in the setting of general practice and primary care
- To promote the development and implementation of research in and into general practice and primary healthcare
- To promote the interests of university departments of general practice by representation on and discussion with interested bodies

---

ANNUAL SCIENTIFIC, GENERAL AND REGIONAL MEETINGS

An annual scientific meeting of the Association is held in July each year, and is the premier UK forum for output from academic departments of general practice. Sessions at these meetings include presentation and discussion of research work and educational or organisational issues relating to members of the Association in their university roles. The 1997 scientific meeting in Dublin was attended by over 400 participants. Papers are invited for submission and are peer-reviewed prior to acceptance for inclusion in the programme. Work is presented in main conference papers, plenary or parallel sessions and as posters for discussion. A selection of conference abstracts are published in the peer-reviewed journal *Family Practice*.

The Annual General Meeting (AGM) takes place during the Annual Scientific Meeting (ASM) and allows for presentation of the Executive's Annual Report for discussion and approval by the membership. Other matters are discussed as appropriate, with the opportunity of voting on matters of significance. Election of officers and members of the Executive Committee is presented and ratified at the AGM.

The ASM represents a national conference for academic general practice, but many departments come together with local colleagues to present academic work and facilitate local communication and discussion of regional issues relating to departments. Such meetings are highly successful and provide the opportunity for colleagues to present work in progress, or for newcomers to departments to present work in a non-threatening and supportive academic environment.

WORKING PARTIES AND KEY REPORTS

The AUDGP has produced a number of papers over the years on topics of direct and immediate relevance to the development of academic general practice. A number of these papers have been published in, and are part of the occasional paper series of the Royal College of General Practitioners, and academic GPs have contributed extensively to the Royal College of General Practitioners publications and position papers. The following are examples of working parties and key reports of the AUDGP over the years:

- University departments of general practice and the undergraduate teaching of general practice in the United Kingdom in 1972. Byrne PS (1993) *Journal of the Royal College of General Practitioners.*
- *Undergraduate Medical Education in General Practitioners: Association of University Teachers in General Practice,* United Kingdom and Republic of Ireland. Occasional Paper 28 (1984). Royal College of General Practitioners, London.
- *The Contribution of Academic General Practice to Undergraduate Medical Education.* Occasional Paper 42. Fraser RC and Preston-White E (1988) Royal College of General Practitioners, London.
- *General Practice in the Medical Schools of United Kingdom – 1986. The McKenzie Report.* Howie JGR, Hannay DR and Stephenson JSK (1986) McKenzie Fund.
- *A Career Structure for Academic General Practice. Final report of a working party of the AUDGP.* (1993) Association of University Departments of General Practice.
- The impacts of increased general practice teaching in the undergraduate medical curriculum. Higgs R and Jones RH (1995) *Education for General Practice* **6**: 218–25.

RESEARCH TRAINING AND SUPPORT

Research training programmes are an ongoing feature of many of the departments, with such training aimed at medical undergraduates and postgraduates, research staff working in departments and enrolled students in Masters courses.

The Association also organises a course in research methodology in conjunction with the Royal College of General Practitioners, which is coordinated by the St George's Hospital Medical School Division of General Practice and Primary Care. Practical and theoretical experience is provided with regard to quantitative and qualitative research techniques, data handling and analysis, presentation of research output and research grant application.

Constituent departments exercise an important role in the focusing and co-ordination of a number of research networks. In the South Thames Region, three academic departments of general practice are involved in supporting the South Thames Research Network of 75 practices involved in important local research initiatives. In this capacity, the academic departments provide supervisory, coordinating and advisory expertise to a large number of GPs in the region.

Departments may also have responsibility for the supervision and support of postgraduate students undertaking higher degrees in general practice or primary care disciplines. Concentration of expertise within such departments provides a uniquely valuable resource in supporting such students, as well as in supporting the incumbents of research training fellowships. Day-to-day support is also frequently provided by members of departments to local GPs undertaking their own research programmes.

REPRESENTATION

The Executive has representation from the United Kingdom Conference of postgraduate directors of general practice education and from the Royal College of General Practitioners and is in turn represented on a wide range of national and international bodies of an academic, professional or governmental nature. Principal bodies on which the AUDGP is currently represented include the Conference of Academic Organisations of General Practice, various Department of Health Advisory Groups, the Council and Committees of the Royal College of General Practitioners and the Primary Care Forum (AUDGP, GMSC, RCGP) of the Department of Health. The Association has had detailed input to discussions regarding the service increment for teaching (SIFT/ACT*), the NHS Research & Development Strategy and the Committee of Vice-Chancellors and Principals (CVCP) Task Force on Clinical Academic Careers. The Association presented oral and written evidence to the House of Lords Committee on Science and Technology in conjunction with the RCGP.

---

* The service increment for teaching (SIFT, England and Wales) and the additional cost of teaching (ACT, Scotland) are payments made to National Health Service institutions in recognition of the additional workload created for service clinicians and their hospitals or trusts on account of the impact of undergraduate medical education on service provision. The AUDGP, largely through the contributions of Professors John Walker and John Howie to negotiations over a fifteen year period, has significantly influenced the resourcing of community-based undergraduate medical education.

RESEARCH OUTPUT

The literature of general practice has expanded enormously in the last 20 years. The contribution of GPs associated with academic departments has been diverse and impressive. It is not possible in a publication of this nature to provide anything more than a 'flavour' of the range of current research interests in which academic general practice is involved. The MacKenzie Report of 1986 identified clinical, operational, behavioural and educational research as the main areas encompassed by the range of research activity within university departments of general practice at that time. The following areas are current and recurrent research themes associated with academic general practice/primary care:

- vocational training for general practitioners
- measuring the quality of care
- access to care and the organisation of services
- stress among GPs
- prevention of disease and health promotion
- drug prescribing, adherence and patients' views on medication
- understanding patients' views of health and illness
- identifying factors influencing clinical behaviour and decision making
- evaluation of new health technologies.

The AUDGP is a national organisation with representative and advisory functions. The Association has input from a wide range of professional clinicians, teachers and researchers from a variety of disciplines represented in university departments of general practice/primary care. Recent years have seen considerable expansion in both the membership and influence of this academic organisation. Involvement in national negotiations regarding the financing and structure of teaching and research in primary care along with the close relationship between the membership and the executive means that this organisation is uniquely placed to influence the development and delivery of primary care in coming years.

REFERENCES

1. Freeman GK (1997) *London Academic Trainee Scheme. Second Annual Report 1996–97.* University of London, London.

2. Fraser RH, Campbell JL, Hill A *et al.* (1993) *A Career Structure for Academic General Practice.* AUDGP, London.

12

The National Primary Care Research and Development Centre and issues at the R&D interface

Brenda Leese, Jackie Bailey and Ann Mahon

INTRODUCTION

The National Primary Care Research and Development Centre (NPCRDC) is a multidisciplinary centre established in 1995 as a collaboration between the Universities of Manchester, York and Salford. NPCRDC is funded by the Department of Health, to undertake a 10-year research and development programme relating to primary healthcare in the UK.

WHAT ARE THE AIMS OF NPCRDC?

The aims of NPCRDC are set out in its annual report for 1996–7[1] as:

- conducting research on primary care
- disseminating research findings to a wide range of audiences
- supporting the development of primary care
- informing primary healthcare policy
- developing and supporting research capacity in primary healthcare.

Table 12.1   Key policy and strategy documents relating to primary care

1994	*Developing NHS Purchasing and GP Fundholding: towards a primary care-led NHS.* EL(94)79[2] introduced total purchasing and other models of fundholding into the NHS
1996	*Priorities and Planning Guidance for the NHS: 1997/1998*[3] gave medium-term priority to work towards the development of a primary care-led NHS, in which decisions about the purchasing and provision of healthcare are taken as close to patients as possible
1996	*Primary Care: the future*[4] reported the results of a consultation exercise on how services in primary healthcare should be developed and sets out the principles of good primary care – quality, fairness, accessibility, responsiveness and efficiency
1996	*Primary Care: the future: choice and opportunity*[5] concerned wider contractual choice, including salaried GPs, practice-based contracts and a unified General Medical Services and Hospital and Community Health Services budget
1996	*Primary Care: the future: delivering the future*[6] described practical proposals to improve primary care, focusing on developing partnerships, professional knowledge, patient and carer involvement and choice, distribution and use of resources, workforce and premises, and better organisation
1997	*NHS (Primary Care) Act* allowed the piloting of different methods for delivering general medical services – Primary Care Act Pilots (PCAPs)
1997	*The New NHS: modern, dependable.*[7] Introduced Primary Care Groups when fundholding is discontinued

WHY IS NPCRDC NEEDED?

In recent years primary care has become central to UK healthcare policy with a series of White Papers and an Act of Parliament which effectively removed many barriers to innovation in primary care organisation (Table 12.1) This policy shift has been accompanied by national and regional research and development strategies, as well as other policy initiatives, which promote the links between research and development within the NHS.

These policy changes are concerned with a number of key issues of considerable relevance to the shaping of primary care services for the 21st century. These issues include: developing new types of primary care organisations able to respond to local needs; actively involving local communities in shaping priorities in health; responding to the changing skills within primary healthcare teams; meeting recruitment and retention challenges in primary care; emphasising the importance of quality of care; developing new arrangements for managing the boundaries between secondary and social care; and developing evidence-based healthcare, management and service development. The NPCRDC research and development programme reflects these key issues.

THE NPCRDC RESEARCH PROGRAMME

This is centred around five main themes.

1 Population health, need and demand for care

This area of the Centre's programme aims to understand the factors shaping the relationship between health, need and demand for care. Delivering a service which is acceptable, responsive and efficient requires an understanding of primary care which incorporates patients' experience of illness and use of services. Better understanding of the actions taken by people in managing their illnesses will enable better management of demand by providing services which complement self and family care.

2 Commissioning, provider organisations and service delivery in primary care

This theme is concerned with: the relationships between contracting and commissioning, the organisations providing primary care and the services which are delivered; the role of patients in shaping both the commissioning/contracting process and the provider organisations; and innovations in primary care and their diffusion to areas of high health need and poor healthcare provision.

3 Workforce and professional roles

This area will contribute to developing a coordinated approach to workforce planning, including reducing inequities in service provision. It aims to identify: how skills should be distributed within primary care teams to maximise cost-effectiveness, patient satisfaction and professional morale; how desired changes in skill mix can best be achieved; and how a better match can be achieved between workforce distribution and population needs, particularly in deprived areas.

4 Quality in primary healthcare

This area of the Centre's programme focuses on three key perspectives of quality: those of health professionals, health authority managers and patients. The aim is to develop indicators of high-quality care which will be easy to apply and where there will be broad agreement that they represent valid measures of quality. Subsequently, this work will seek to identify how quality standards can be used to help practitioners to improve the services which they provide.

5 Boundaries and interfaces between primary care, secondary care and social care

This theme aims to identify the effect of shifts between primary and secondary care, and between health and social services, on both primary and community health services and on patients. It is also concerned with how services can be appropriately organised and coordinated across organisational and professional boundaries to meet the needs of people with complex and/or long-term needs, and how the organisation of services can better reflect the choices of service users and informal carers.

THE CORE VALUES

The programme described above is underpinned by a set of core values which emphasise the Centre's belief in:

- *equitable provision of primary healthcare* by examining issues related to inequities in health and healthcare provision
- *patient-led healthcare* by helping the NHS to be more responsive to the people who use it
- *multidisciplinary primary healthcare* by examining how a wide range of disciplines can work together to provide comprehensive, accessible and cost-effective primary care
- *quality and cost-effectiveness* by increasing knowledge of services which are cost-effective, to develop and disseminate quality standards and to support the development of knowledge-based primary healthcare
- *research-based service development* by a commitment to bridging the gap between academic research and service development, and promoting research based service development in primary care.

REGIONAL RESEARCH ADVISORY SERVICE

The Centre is committed to bridging the gap between academic research and service development, to promote research-based service development in primary care and to promote research awareness and skills of NHS staff. To this latter end, the Centre is funded by the NHSE North West Regional Office to provide a free Research Advisory Service to any NHS employee within the North West Region wanting assistance with health services research and development, particularly related to primary care. The majority of clients are primary care professionals and managers, and in the past year the Centre has served 177 clients. The nature of the services provided to clients is highly varied and includes: assistance with the design and conduct of research and development projects; advice and assistance with conducting electronic and other literature searches; provision of research intelligence to health commissioners; serving on steering groups of local development projects; supervision of Regional Research Training Fellows; advising on the development of local primary care research networks; and serving on grant-giving research and development committees.

THE DISSEMINATION STRATEGY

The Centre's aim is to disseminate research findings and promote service development based on sound evidence of effectiveness, efficiency and appropriateness. To this end, a dissemination team has been established at the Centre. The results of research and development in primary care are disseminated to four distinct audiences:

- policy makers at national, regional and local levels
- managers and health professionals in the NHS
- the academic and scientific research community
- users of primary care and organisations which represent users.

The types of outputs are designed to reflect the differing needs of the various audiences. The academic and scientific research community are likely to require detailed outputs for critical analysis and comment, whereas managers and professionals may find summaries and general articles sufficient for their need to apply research findings in their own specific environment. Readily accessible articles in the popular media are designed primarily for health professionals, users and carers and those without access to the more specialised publications. Conferences aim to promote discussion and comment from a wide range of academics, professionals and managers. Table 12.2 shows the various types of NPCRDC outputs and their target audiences.

THE DEVELOPMENT STRATEGY

Development is one of the key objectives of the Centre and takes a number of forms, ranging from contributions to organisational development of primary care

Table 12.2 NPCRDC target audiences and typical outputs

Target audience	Typical output
Academic and scientific research community	Books and articles in peer-reviewed journals
Professionals working in primary healthcare	Articles in professional journals and trade magazines
Managers and health professionals	Executive summaries of research findings
Research community, managers, professionals and policy makers	Briefing papers and research reports summarising research findings and implications for practice
Research community, professionals and policy makers	Discussion papers to contribute to debates around primary care policy, practice and research
Professionals, users and organisations representing users and carers	Media briefings and press releases for a wide range of professional and popular media
Academic research community	Presentations of research findings to academic and scientific meetings
Managers and professionals	Contributions to local and national meetings of NHS managers and professionals to inform, promote discussion and facilitate development
Wider research community, professionals and managers	Organisation of Centre conferences, workshops and seminars around research and development themes within primary care
All groups	Website information (under development)

and research, to longer-term projects. In February 1997, NPCRDC launched a new development partnership with the King's Fund Development Centre, designed to support primary care development in the pilot sites established as a result of the *NHS (Primary Care) Act 1997* (Table 12.1).

Partnerships have been established with eight 'demonstration sites' with the aim of commissioning comprehensive primary care and supporting these developments with applied evaluative research. These plans have been set out in detail in an NPCRDC/King's Fund Discussion paper.[8] This development proposal contains a description of the policy context for the forthcoming changes, a model of the development process, how the demonstration sites will be supported, details of some of the research questions and a timetable for a four-and-a-half-year programme of development, research and dissemination.

The aim is for the small group of pilot partnership sites to provide opportunities to demonstrate what it is possible to achieve and for the associated evaluative research to provide sound evidence with which to identify good practice. Over the lifetime of the project, the aim will be to provide demonstrations of good practice in a variety of circumstances. The demonstration sites will focus on the commissioning of comprehensive primary care services, and the development of new forms of primary care provider organisations. They highlight the interest within the Centre in evaluating experimental arrangements in primary care that would be of interest to a wider national audience.

The Centre's extensive programme of research and development will increasingly enable us to make important contributions to the knowledge base necessary to support development in primary care, while at the same time, the new service developments will provide opportunities for partnerships in development and research.

THE INTERFACE BETWEEN RESEARCH AND DEVELOPMENT

Two projects from the Centre's portfolio of projects can be used to illustrate work at the interface between research and development. These are the evaluation of total purchasing pilots and the evaluation of Primary Care Resource Centres.

The evaluation of total purchasing pilots (TPP) project is managed by the King's Fund and is a consortium which includes researchers from the Universities of Southampton, Bristol and Edinburgh, as well as from NPCRDC.[9] The Centre staff are responsible for collecting 'core' data from 14 of the 53 projects in North West, Trent and Northern and Yorkshire Regions. This has involved conducting face-to-face interviews with key stakeholders – lead GP, site manager, health authority lead, and representatives from providers and social services – at each TPP. This has been augmented by the collection of relevant documentation, such as purchasing plans, from each TPP to enable a picture to be built up of, not only what is to be purchased, but also how the TPP is developing and creating the climate for success. The research is therefore taking place in a changing and developing environment which has effects on the ways in which the research is conducted and the conclusions which can be drawn, as discussed in more detail below.

The evaluation of Primary Care Resource Centres (PCRCs) was commissioned by the former North West Regional Health Authority (NWRHA).[10] The evaluation focused on a major capital investment strategy involving the construction of 17 PCRCs across northwest England at a cost of £19 million. The development of four centres was studied in detail, using interviews with key stakeholders, observation at key meetings, documentary analysis and collection of cost data and centre users' views. The study concluded that major capital developments like this needed considerable time to bring together different organisations and local people and to identify new streams of revenue funding to support new service developments. Good project management and the active involvement of health authorities, GPs and local communities are also essential if capital developments in primary care are to extend services and improve health and wellbeing in deprived urban areas. This formative evaluation was complemented by two service development workshops for those involved in developing PCRCs in the North West Region.

ISSUES ARISING FROM RESEARCH AT THE INTERFACE BETWEEN RESEARCH AND DEVELOPMENT

There are three major components to a service and policy evaluation. The *structural* component focuses on the levels and organisation of service inputs, while a *process* evaluation is concerned with the way service outputs are developed and accessed by various groups of stakeholders, for example, patients, managers and health professionals. The third component of an evaluation relates to *outcomes,* whereby the measurable effects of service outputs, service use or other interventions can be assessed. Both the PCRCs evaluation and the TPP project used a 'process evaluation' approach, employing stakeholder-based and case study methods.

Process evaluations can be defined as:

> *... aimed at elucidating and understanding the internal dynamics of program operations. They focus on the following kinds of questions: What are the factors that come together to make this program what it is? What are the strengths and weaknesses of the program? ... Process evaluations most typically require a detailed description of program operations ... The 'process' focus in an evaluation implies an emphasis on how a product or outcome is produced rather than looking at the product itself; that is, it is an analysis of the processes whereby a program produces the results it does. Process evaluation is developmental, descriptive, continuous, flexible, and inductive.*[11]

Outcome (or summative) evaluation has tended to dominate the field of health services research. This approach to evaluation can be used to assess efficiency, effectiveness, equity, acceptability, accessibility, appropriateness, accountability, choice and so on. However, these global or all embracing concepts do not lend themselves readily to empirical investigation or measurement. Furthermore, following the introduction of a policy initiative, it often takes many years before tangible changes can be identified and measured. Even when such a timescale has elapsed, the problem of attribution, namely identifying the precise factors that lead to a particular outcome, are such that it is often extremely difficult, if not impossible, to demonstrate cause-and-effect relationships. An outcome-based approach to evaluation requires the existence of pre-determined outcome criteria. However, it is often the case in policy initiatives that the appropriate criteria for evaluation emerge gradually, as the policy initiative itself evolves and so, in contrast to outcome evaluation, process evaluation is not dependent on pre-determined criteria for evaluation and, indeed, its strength lies in its sensitivity to the evolutionary nature of policy interpretation and implementation.

The following sections explore some of the issues which were raised by the two studies described above. Many of these issues are not exclusive to process evaluation and might well be of relevance to other evaluation models.

RATIONALE FOR THE STUDY DESIGN AND METHODS

Primary Care Resource Centres (PCRCs)

An initial descriptive 'mapping' exercise had identified centres open, being built or planned. From this it was found that few centres were fully operational; many were at planning or building stages. This placed constraints on both the scope and the methods of any evaluation. Marked variations in the objectives, funding and organisation of these initiatives were clearly discernible. There were clear differences apparent in the processes being employed in different localities to achieve their objectives. These differences called for early evaluation; there are limits on the extent to which their significance and impact might reliably be reconstructed through later, *post-hoc* evaluation.

Many 'stakeholders' were involved in the planning, funding and management of the centres and in the provision and use of services located or planned within them. These stakeholders included RHA, health authority and/or family health services authority staff; GPs and other members of primary healthcare teams; community health professionals and therapists working within the community; hospital staff whose diagnostic and therapy services might be relocated in the new centres; service users, potential users and members of local community groups; local authority staff whose services would be located in the centre; and the purchasers and providers of other statutory and independent welfare and advice services to be based within a centre. There were likely to be differences between the various stakeholders in the extent to which they agreed with centre goals; in how they interpreted them; and in how they implemented them. Variations both within and between different centres, in the objectives and criteria for success of the various stakeholders, were also likely. Therefore the evaluation needed to be pluralistic[12] in the sense that these different perspectives are acknowledged and incorporated into the research design. Because of the diversity of the people involved in PCRC development, a stakeholder approach was adopted.[13]

Total Purchasing Pilots (TPPs)

The study of the process of setting up and operating total purchasing included, among other things, an assessment of their aims and objectives and their achievements. Initially it was assumed that total purchasing would develop as a straightforward extension to fundholding, but it soon became apparent that this was not the case. Total purchasing was introduced into the NHS in 1994 following an Executive Letter[2] which included no details about what the pilot projects were expected to achieve. The absence of any stated aims and objectives nationally meant that these would have to evolve from within the projects themselves, as products of their particular approaches to the interpretation and implementation of total purchasing. Quite clearly this requires a process-based approach to evaluation. As in the case of PCRCs, TPPs were characterised by the involvement of a large number of stakeholders; GPs, project managers, health authorities, providers and social services.

SOME PROBLEMS AND CHALLENGES ASSOCIATED WITH PROCESS EVALUATIONS

In this section we will briefly look at some of the problems and challenges encountered during our process evaluations.

- *Stakeholder-based methods:* there are problems associated with the stakeholder method, some of which were encountered during both the PCRC and TPP studies. There are methodological issues surrounding the validity and reliability of multistakeholder perspectives. There are possible tensions between different stakeholders and potential conflicts of interest. There is also the risk of stakeholders attempting to control or influence the evaluation in a particular direction. Often in such process evaluations differences in accounts reflect differences in opinion, experience and perceptions. How a researcher deals with such differences raises some fundamental questions about validity and reliability but it also reinforces the relevance and appropriateness of the stakeholder-based approach to evaluation.
- *Confidentiality and negotiating access:* an essential step in the evaluation process adopted in the PCRC study was offering stakeholders the opportunity to comment on the draft study reports concerning accuracy, coverage and fairness

of interpretation. The anonymity of respondents was, as far as possible, protected. Respondents were given a written or verbal undertaking that their accounts would be treated with the utmost confidentiality. This undertaking included a guarantee not to name locations or individuals and the promise that respondents would be able to see relevant sections of written reports before publication, to ensure that they were accurate. There were two reasons for undertaking this checking process. In the course of identifying potential study sites and negotiating access, some key stakeholders expressed considerable anxiety about collaborating with the evaluation because of the confidential nature of financial and business planning documents and the sensitivity of some of the negotiations between purchasers and potential service providers. These anxieties reflected some of the commercial sensitivities which are increasingly associated with the internal market, where business interests are likely to have a growing impact on the development of primary care. The commitment to allow respondents a right of veto over the reported research material was a way of acknowledging and responding to these anxieties and formed part of the confidentiality agreement negotiated with local stakeholders. Furthermore, over the six-month fieldwork period, many details of the proposed PCRCs changed considerably: proposed services were withdrawn; other new services were introduced; key stakeholders moved in and out of posts; above all, perceptions and opinions shifted with the passage of time and the progress of events. Moreover, the NWRHA's PCRC initiative as a whole evolved, as new procedures for bidding for funding were developed.

- *Policy process:* the total purchasing evaluation presented a number of challenges to the evaluation team, and those relating to the policy process will be briefly considered here. The absence of a blueprint for total purchasing has been discussed earlier in this chapter. While this laissez faire approach to policy making encourages innovation, it can present considerable challenges to evaluators attempting to come to some decision about the relative merits of the policy since the concept evolves gradually and the method of evaluation must be appropriate to capture this. The policy context was further complicated by national and local policy changes that inevitably had a knock-on effect on how total purchasing would develop in the different pilot projects. This included the formation of new health authorities as well as various local provider reconfigurations. Both the ambiguous nature of total purchasing and the national and local changes that accompanied its implementation presented considerable challenges to the evaluation team in terms of identifying criteria of success, and this has been the focus of much debate among the research team.[14] There is no single and definitive approach to defining success and, indeed, at least four distinct perspectives have been identified: the official perspective, the academic perspective, the viewpoint of opinion leaders and product champions and the views of the stakeholders themselves. A further approach is currently being developed by the research team and involves the identification of a number of outcome measures based on the findings of the process evaluation to date.

- *The role of the researcher in process evaluations:* the role of the researcher in process evaluations is less clear cut than in outcome evaluations. This was certainly the case in the total purchasing evaluation where, as well as interviewer or observer, the researcher also assumed the role of information-giver, confidant and facilitator. The appropriateness of assuming multiple roles is clearly an issue of debate, not least because of the implications for the validity of the research findings but also because of the additional responsibility and potential for conflict that it introduces.
- *Wider relevance/transferability/generalisability of a local initiative:* the development of PCRCs reflected an explicit strategy within the NWRHA for developing the range and the quality of primary health services. However, there were other initiatives, both within the North West and elsewhere in England, which shared similar features apart from having a single, ear-marked source of capital funding. They also appeared to be more closely grounded in local purchaser, provider or community initiatives, rather than reflecting regional strategic priorities. The evaluation therefore incorporated comparisons of different funding and development strategies. This yielded information which would be helpful to other Regions which may be considering similar capital investment programmes, and to purchasers and providers elsewhere who are considering different local strategies for promoting innovation and development in primary and community health services.

A common perception of the general policy shift towards increasing localisation is that it becomes increasingly difficult to draw general lessons that are of wider relevance to the NHS. This is not, however, the case since local influences and circumstances will often develop and adapt policy initiatives whether they originate from the Department of Health or from the local context. Different models of total purchasing have now been identified and have considerable relevance to current policy debates. The Government's plans for re-organising the NHS include the introduction of Primary Care Groups. The findings from the total purchasing evaluation have both timely and relevant messages for these and other policy developments in the NHS.

FROM RESEARCH TO DISSEMINATION TO PRACTICE?

Evidence-based policy making and service developments are dependent on effective dissemination strategies. In Table 12.2 we summarised NPCRDC's dissemination strategy which identified target audiences and outputs specifically designed to meet their needs. This principle informed our respective dissemination strategies for the projects described above. Whilst the methods employed in process evaluations challenge the conventional outcome-based model built around the scientific paradigm, it requires a commensurate shift in evidence-based management to ensure that the results of policy evaluations are implemented in practice.

REFERENCES

1. National Primary Care Research and Development Centre. Annual Report, 1996–7.

2. NHS Executive (1994) *Developing NHS Purchasing and GP Fundholding: towards a primary care-led NHS.* EL(94)79. Department of Health, London.

3. NHS Executive (1996) *Priorities and Planning Guidance for the NHS: 1997/98.* Department of Health, London.

4. Department of Health (1996) *Primary Care: the future.* Department of Health, London.

5. Department of Health (1996) *Primary Care: the future – choice and opportunity.* Department of Health, London.

6. Department of Health (1996) *Primary Care: delivering the future.* Department of Health, London.

7. Department of Health (1997) *The New NHS: modern, dependable.* The Stationery Office, London.

8. Wilkin D, Butler T and Coulter A (1997) *New models of primary care: developing the future.* Discussion Paper 2. National Primary Care Research and Development Centre/ King's Fund.

9. TP-NET (1997) *Total Purchasing: a profile of national pilot projects.* King's Fund, London.

10. Glendinning C, Bailey J, Burkey Y *et al.* (1996) *An evaluation of Primary Care Resource Centres in the North West of England.* NPCRDC Report, University of Manchester.

11. Patton MQ (1987) *How to Use Qualitative Methods in Evaluation.* Sage, London.

12. Smith G and Cantley C (1985) *Assessing Health Care: a study in organisational evaluation.* Open University Press, Milton Keynes.

13. Weiss CA (1983) The stakeholder approach to evaluation: origins and promise. In: AS Bryk (ed) *Stakeholder-based Evaluation.* Jossey-Bass, San Francisco.

14. Mahon A, Leese B, Baxter K *et al.* (1998) *Determining Success Criteria for Total Purchasing Pilots.* TP-NET Working Paper. King's Fund, London.

13

Writing for peer-reviewed journals

Alastair Wright

THE VALUE OF WRITING UP

Every completed piece of general practitioner research deserves to be written up, whether or not it is published. The process of composing a scientific paper and providing references gives further insight on both the research itself and the scientific method. It is part of the continuing self-education needed to understand and use research. Publication in a reputable journal is the next logical step. It gives well-earned personal satisfaction, advances careers and distributes the work widely to others, who may use the findings for their own research or in clinical practice.

Modern science began after the invention of printing. It was printing that made it possible for researchers to become aware of each other's work and to make progress. The computer and the Internet are very much with us and welcome, but reports of the death of printing have been greatly exaggerated. Screens are less portable and much less easy to read than the printed word. The journal, printed on paper, is still alive and well.

SCIENTIFIC JOURNALS AND EVIDENCE-BASED MEDICINE

Medical journals can be classified into two main types: those that publish original research and those that do not. The former are called primary or 'record' journals because they record scientific advances. The second group, information journals, do not normally publish original work but rather digests or features based on other peoples' original work. Journals of information are very important for keeping up to date but it is vital that their contents are based on sound, reliable research work. Their job is to summarise the evidence for working clinicians. Both types of journal have a place in supporting evidence-based medicine, but the research papers in journals of record, such as *British Journal of General Practice* or *Family Practice, are* the evidence for evidence-based general practice. This does not mean that there is published evidence for every treatment or that clinical judgement and experience are in any way devalued. Clinicians should be aware of the written evidence, able to assess its value critically and reflect on it in relation to patients seen day by day. Otherwise clinical practice deteriorates over time.

It is vitally important for general practice to have journals of record to publish research advances in general practice as distinct from republishing work from specialist disciplines. Research is fundamentally a process of personal education which is also of direct benefit to patients as it promotes the professional development of the doctor by improving critical and problem-solving skills, which in turn enhance job satisfaction. For general practitioners as a group there is a need not only for research in general practice but for research *into* general practice itself.

Peer review: distilling research into evidence

Journals of record select articles by peer review, a process that is not confined to medicine but which is common to academic publishing worldwide. The aim is that papers are treated consistently according to internationally accepted rules, so that publication depends on perceived scientific quality and relevance to the appropriate discipline rather than commercial considerations. Papers are assessed independently by experts and published according to the conventions of the scientific world.

Printed journals are important for the dissemination of technical knowledge and ideas to doctors but journals which are peer reviewed do more than distribute information. The process of peer review involves sifting through huge amounts of reported research, distilling it to manageable levels and in the process screening out faulty results or poorly conducted studies. In this way clinical practice can and should be based on reliable evidence that has been assessed carefully. It also helps select which research is published by giving papers a priority ranking based on a knowledge of the literature. There is more to a journal than the individual articles: it is the package that lends credibility to the contents and helps the reader zero in on material that is relevant and worthwhile to him or her.

Peer review is not without its critics and there have recently been calls for the process to be more open.[1] It is criticised as being biased towards experienced researchers and resulting in papers 'doctored' to reflect reviewers' opinions. Delaying publication for peer review is claimed to blunt the 'cutting edge' of progress, but the traditional journal publishing cycle is a check-and-balance system that separates the wheat from the chaff. Patients can be caused unnecessary distress when speculation at medical conferences is reported on television or at press conferences as if it were a proven advance in treatment. The process of peer review is not perfect but it is still the best we have.

THE BONES OF AN ARTICLE

In medicine, it is expected that research papers will be presented in a standard format, which makes life easier both for editors and readers. Most medical journals follow the standards of the International Committee of Medical Journal Editors,[2] commonly called the Vancouver Group as this body grew out of a meeting of medical editors in Vancouver in 1978. Authors are well advised to follow these guidelines. Details specific to an individual journal will be found in a section containing information for authors. Papers can be handled more quickly if authors read and follow the house style before sending in a paper.

Success in scientific writing depends on getting a good study and then applying the rules of academic writing. Articles describing clinical studies may have become increasingly sophisticated, but the fundamentals have not changed. It is exceptionally easy *not* to say what you mean so that a good study can be let down by the writing. Reviewers may ask themselves if lack of attention to detail in the writing indicates lack of attention to detail in the research.

Editors expect a research paper to answer four fundamental questions: why I started, what I did, what I found and what it means. These translate into the conventional headings: Introduction, Methods, Results and Discussion (Box 13.1). The sections are interrelated: the methods should be capable of answering the research questions posed in the introduction and conclusions should be drawn directly from the data presented in the results section. After a straight read the reviewer will check through this traditional structure for a scientific paper before analysing the work in detail. You should check your own projects along the same lines. People still put results in the discussion and some methods in the results or even results in the introduction and this confuses and alarms reviewers, editors and readers alike.

Box 13.1 Structure of a scientific paper

- Introduction: why I started
- Method: what I did
- Results: what I found
- Discussion: what it means

The Introduction should give the background to the paper, showing that there is a gap in knowledge which your research is about to answer and then stating what you need to establish, that is: your aims. Here you should introduce the references (but not too many) to previous research in the same field. References should be directly relevant to your research questions and should not be copied thoughtlessly from a computer search.

A clear Methods section is vital to the credibility of your results. Established research methods or well known questionnaires can be covered by giving a reference, but methods that have been published but are not well known should be briefly described. New or substantially modified methods need a fuller description and you should give reasons for using them and your evaluation of their limitations. Provide a concise account of statistical methods here, including references if they are unusual and specify, but do not elaborate on, the computer program used in the analysis.

The Results section answers the question 'what did you find?'. The text will usually summarise only the main findings with the detail of the data being presented as tables or figures. The main difficulty in composing this section is often not what to put in but what to leave out.

The Discussion gives the author the opportunity to say what he or she makes of the findings as he or she answers the question 'what does it mean?'. This section can highlight the new and important aspects of the research and relate it to other relevant studies. Limitations of the research should be acknowledged and conclusions should not go beyond what is supported by the data, though it is reasonable to state new hypotheses if they are acknowledged as such.

WHAT REVIEWERS AND EDITORS LOOK FOR

Reviewers provide advice to the editor, who makes the final decision on publication, sometimes aided by a 'hanging committee' or similar group. They are usually asked whether the work is sufficiently original to merit publication and for their views on scientific quality, clinical importance and relevance to the readership. Often the journal will supply guidelines or a checklist to assist in assessing the paper. Most journals ask for detailed criticism of the paper to be typed on a sheet to be passed on to the author and for recommendations and any confidential comments to the editor on a separate page.

Many journals do not have enough space to publish all the papers recommended by referees so editors must make a choice from those papers of acceptable quality on the basis of topicality, reader interest and importance for practice (Box 13.2). Papers that provide new findings on a common disease are very attractive to editors, especially where improved management or prognosis can be demonstrated. The editor has also to think beyond the individual paper to consider the mixture of papers and articles in any one issue.

> **Box 13.2   Publishing questions**
>
> Is the work:
> - New: giving new information or insight on the subject?
> - True: scientifically reliable, conclusions supported by the data in the paper?
> - Important: clinically as well as statistically significant?
> - Suitable: or too specialised or peripheral for the main readership?

WHAT AUTHORS SHOULD LOOK FOR

Authors should first consider a journal that is likely to be interested in the subject of the paper. Other factors to take into account are whether the work would be indexed and included in research databases, how likely it would be to be quoted by other researchers and how quickly it might be quoted. The answers to the latter questions depend principally on the interest and quality of the research work but also on the standing in its field of the journal publishing the paper.

Index Medicus, published monthly by the National Library of Medicine in the USA, contains citations to the biomedical journal literature and aims to provide 'access to the highest quality and most important biomedical and health sciences journals published throughout the world'. For general practice/primary care only ten journals are accepted. Within those journals original articles are indexed, as well as letters, editorials and some articles that are thought to have substantive contents.

A citation is the formal acknowledgement by an author of previously published research and is recorded in the list of references accompanying the paper. Citations are therefore an important indicator of how frequently present-day researchers are using the journal literature. The annual *Journal Citation Reports*[3] give comparative data on 6000 of the world's leading journals. Authors can thus compare journals in their field of interest with regard to the average number of citations to articles published in the journal (Impact Factor) and the average number of times the journal's articles are cited in the same year they are published (Immediacy Index). In this way authors can have some idea how likely their article is to be noticed by other researchers if published in a particular journal and also how quickly it is likely to be noticed.

THE SECRETS OF GETTING PUBLISHED

Later in this chapter Joe Kai gives clear practical advice on drafting, revising and writing effectively. Having done your market research and designed the paper for your target journal do not neglect the final tasks of quality control or polish and packaging (Box 13.3). At this stage some authors run out of steam at the final

---

Box 13.3   Preparing for publication

- Market research
- Design for target
- Quality control
- Polish and packaging

---

hurdle and send in a potentially good paper with a poor summary and a mis-leading makeshift title.

Your cherished paper should be accompanied by a letter pointing out, as appropriate, the topicality of the subject, the originality of the findings or the clinical relevance of the results. A compliments slip initialled by your secretary suggests that you have run out of steam – or enthusiasm. Try not to send the submission with a dog-eared summary in the format of the journal that has just turned down the paper. Journal editors will look beyond the typescript to assess the quality of the work but a well-written, cleanly typed paper makes a good impression on both editors and referees. Careless, shoddy presentation may make reviewers think that the research work may have been careless and shoddy as well. Please read the instructions for authors – this will save you time. A crisp, reader-friendly style is ideal but you should not sacrifice clarity or accuracy: scientific prose is not meant primarily for works of the imagination. It is worthwhile to look carefully at all your adjectives and adverbs to check that they add worthwhile meaning. This is what subeditors do. Be careful that you say what you mean. Lastly, remember that authors and editors have a common interest in providing interesting and sound scientific papers for readers.

Putting research to paper

Joe Kai

Before you start a project, writing a paper can sound straightforward. It seems to be a simple matter of reporting what had transpired. But as you reach the point when you actually ought to do so, it can seem more daunting. Alastair Wright has provided some of the theory and clear guidelines from an editor's perspective. In what follows, I offer some more personal experiences about writing papers for publication. I hope this gives a flavour of what the process can be like and perhaps a few practical suggestions. I hope too that those considering doing some research or reporting their work may be encouraged to start writing and to see their hard labours bear fruit. I have come to think that it's worth it – after a while.

THE ART OF PROCRASTINATION

So, finally, all those project delays and setbacks are over. The finished data lies before you. They may even be fully analysed and interpreted. Unfortunately there now follows a long delay. Why? Because you do your level best to avoid starting to write up. Surely there are still references to chase before you can really begin? Or could there be more data to collect? Perhaps you should wait till after you attend that workshop because doubtless you will learn something crucial to enhancing your paper. Alternatively there's the moral high ground argument. Your neglected patients need you. Not to mention your overworked practice colleagues. And anyway your partners' holidays are all overlapping in the next two months and the practice could be busy.... If you aren't a 'completer-finisher', how do you avoid the often unconscious but irresistible urge to put off writing a paper?

First, do not swiftly move on to some entirely new activity which you justify as important because it will be clearly related to your, as yet unwritten, research. Second, do not suddenly be overcome by diffidence. This is where you decide that the work you've completed is actually not up to much and barely worth mentioning in conversation, let alone committing to print and the scrutiny of your peers. Shirking the task like this is surely even worse than fear of censure. Moreover, no one will believe you. *Mea culpa* to both these cowardly strategies. There is much to gain, and if you have conducted a project then you acquired certain responsibilities when you did so. You need to give your current work the attention it deserves now!

A MORAL IMPERATIVE?

The value of writing up is highlighted earlier in the chapter. You also have obligations to write up your work: an obligation to those the research was intended to help; an obligation to those you involved – be they study participants, your co-workers or your sponsors; an obligation to your colleagues in the wider healthcare or research community to ensure they learn from your experience; and of course an obligation to do the work and yourself justice. Not to mention friends and family that have put up with several preceding months of worthy monologue about your project. If you feel any happier, or perhaps take this all as read, you must now ask yourself why *you* want to have your work published. If you are not absolutely clear, then perhaps you should leave the job to someone else. Once you can answer why (self-advancement is not only permitted but entirely legitimate here), then you can set about the task ahead with alacrity.

GETTING STARTED

This is the most difficult hurdle for me and for many others. You may be someone who does not have the immediacy of clinical service pressures, but for many in primary care this is not the case. There will always be other things you can do in the time available. You need to make the time to be able to sit down and put pen to paper or, more likely, fingers to keyboard. This may mean, for example, ensuring you allot a certain period of a certain day each week that is devoted just to writing up. You may need to be ruthless about not doing something else so that you have made this space. Further delicate negotiations with family or partner may also be required. Fail to do this and it's amazing how the weeks, then months, fly by with nothing but good intentions to show for it.

Next, be clear about how you are going to use your valuable time. At this stage, it is customary for me to decide I will plan, draft and revise a paper in a hopelessly optimistic timespan. Set stages and objectives you know are easily achievable, for example re-acquainting yourself with the background literature in one stage and planning the key points for the introduction to your paper in another period. Attach timescales to these stages that are clearly realistic (probably months rather than weeks), and assess how you are doing regularly.

Box 13.4   Starting out

- Beware the art of procrastination
- Make and protect the time
- Set yourself realistic, achievable objectives

WRITING CLEARLY AND EFFECTIVELY

A helpful first step is to sit back and think what it is you really want to say. Having got this far in completing your research, this question can be a searching and sometimes disconcerting one. It means deciding first, what is the key message from your work? Second, who are you writing for? Third, ensuring you convey your message as simply as possible to your intended audience.

Distilling a clear message from your experiences or findings can be more challenging than you think. There are often many points you can make that may be eligible for emphasis. Try and resist the temptation to underline all of them. Focus instead on highlighting one or two key messages you want readers to take away. I try to play around with all the different messages I can think of before drafting an article. I then isolate up to three which seem the most important, interesting and relevant. As you are often too 'close' to the work, it can be helpful to present colleagues from the journal audience with the list of potential points you have and ask them to select the most appropriate.

Next, be clear and concise. Do not feel that if you are writing a 'scientific' article it should be presented using erudite and technical text. Your primary aim is to communicate. You might start writing thinking you won't have enough to say, but this rarely turns out to be the case. Invariably I find it is much harder to leave material out than it is to include it. If it is not essential to the message can it be cut? It is worth reading the tabloid press, not for the news content or searching commentary, but to grasp the highly effective style of communication. Each article will usually present just one message, using short words to form short, pithy sentences.

Box 13.5   Communicating effectively

- What do you really want to say?
- Match the message to your potential audience
- Write simply and concisely
- If it's not essential then leave it out

DRAFTING THE ARTICLE

The standard, structured format for most papers, what to include in the different sections and what editors look for was referred to earlier. It should be said that this traditional format has yet to be revised to allow effective presentation of qualitative research in the major healthcare journals. I have found it productive to operate a few rules so that an article looks (and hopefully is) interesting and worth reading.

Think about how you would approach and read another article for the first time. People see the title first – does it grab you? Is your curiosity sparked sufficiently to read on? Invest time in choosing a title. Readers then turn to the summary or abstract. This is crucial – if people are struck by the carefully honed, clear messages this contains, they may read on. More likely they will actually skip to the 'what it means' section – the discussion – and in particular to the first paragraphs. Here, as far as possible, I try and capture in the first sentence or two the significance of the work or the principal finding. This needs to be done with care so that you do not inappropriately exaggerate the importance of the work. Almost in the same breath, show some humility. Discuss any limitations of your work and how they might have been, or could be, negotiated.

INVITE YOUR FRIENDS

The draft is done. Do not falter now and just send it off. Getting comments on your draft is invaluable, but choose carefully. I usually ask a range of colleagues for help. This includes those who might be part of the target audience; people likely to have entirely different perspectives to your own; and those who will not be reluctant to give constructive criticism. Finally, ask people who are far removed from the area under discussion, for example non-health professionals, friends and family to read it. If from a lay perspective the article is interesting and readable then you are on the right tracks. Limit the number you involve in this process or you can end up with so many contradictory comments that redrafting becomes a nightmare. Redrafting, however, is a fact of writing up, and draft after draft at that. This can be a highly frustrating process. Sometimes I have found my fourth draft bears only a passing resemblance to my first!

SUBMITTING THE ARTICLE

Alastair Wright draws attention to the importance of presentation of the manuscript and running a final check on your paper. Do not then underestimate the importance of a covering letter to the editor. Other than the article itself this is the only opportunity you have to get his or her ear and put your case. Your letter needs to be short (certainly less than one side) but must include why you feel the article is going to be of relevance and importance to the journal's audience. Editors are also interested in topicality, so refer to this, if appropriate. In particular, draw attention to any originality of your work, a key criterion for publication, for example new findings, an unexplored topic or use of a particular approach in your study setting.

COPING WITH REJECTION

All that work and in a few brief words your hopes are dashed. Having overcome fleeting misanthropy directed at the editor or reviewer (who clearly didn't understand your work at all), get it out of your system. Leave some space by all means. This is a demoralising time. However, do not then rehearse the delay tactics mentioned above. You need to reassess. Remember your obligations. You may have suffered a loss of confidence. You may even persuade yourself that your work is clearly unworthy and insignificant. But all work should find an audience and be disseminated. It adds to a body of knowledge and experience. Those researchers who publish prolifically will tell you they receive many more rejections than acceptances. Their advice is to keep going till you appear in print. If you have been provided with reviewers' comments, then do at least see if they have a point. Most reviewers try to be constructive. Is it worth revising the article before resubmitting to another journal? If you do, bear in mind any new audience and style of the journal.

If, despite revisions, you keep getting rejections then remember that peer-reviewed journals are only one of many outlets for your work. Cynics may argue, perhaps with more truth than academics might be prepared to admit, that research in peer-reviewed journals has minimal impact on real life. The same may not be true of the many professional educational publications. Reporting your article in more populist form may be just as effective in meeting some of your obligations to write up and may well have more practical impact.

ON BEING PUBLISHED

If the Gods are smiling on you – and sometimes it really is a matter of luck – then enjoy it while it lasts. Fortunately this is usually a long time because having been accepted for publication there will be a delay of anywhere between three months to a year before your article actually appears. However, the journal will usually require revisions in line with reviewers' and editor's comments. Do not be afraid to discuss queries with the editor's team and negotiate revisions that are problematic.

IS IT WORTH IT?

There are sacrifices to make, yes. Your family, friends and colleagues will live through your travails, but also hopefully your success. Those who have been doing more service work in your absence will forever be owed that odd late house call on a Friday evening. Guilt is a powerful thing. Rewards? Well, fame and presumably fortune for some. More importantly, you have discharged certain responsibilities as a researcher. For the individual, the process of writing up un-doubtedly forces you to think and reflect more effectively on what you have done. This can only be good, and if you learn a few skills and something about yourself on the way, so much the better. Finally, while you won't really want to admit it, everyone enjoys the approbation of their peers. Go on, have a go.

REFERENCES

1. Smith R (1997) Peer review: reform or revolution? *BMJ.* **315**: 759–60.

2. International Committee of Medical Journal Editors (1997) *Uniform Requirements for Manuscripts Submitted to Biomedical Journals,* 5th edn. ICMJE, Philadelphia, PA.

3. Institute for Scientific Information (1995) *Journal Citation Reports.* 1995 Science edition. Institute for Scientific Information, Philadelphia, PA.

FURTHER READING

Albert T (1997) *Winning the Publications Game: how to get published without neglecting your patients.* Radcliffe Medical Press, Oxford.

Fraser J (1997) *How to Publish in Biomedicine: 500 tips for success.* Radcliffe Medical Press, Oxford.

14

Going it alone: a view from the grassroots

Norman Beale

ONE-HORSE TOWN

There used to be a parking bay in the shadow of the north wall of Calne Town Hall. We stopped there, in the first few days of 1976, to look at the instructions for finding the senior partner's house. In fact, we found ourselves gaping at the huge and hugely unattractive building opposite. C & T Harris Co. Ltd, Bacon Curers [By Appointment] were, my wife and I would learn over lunch, *the* commercial enterprise, and the social hub, of Calne. A small butcher's shop opened in 1770 had grown backwards and upwards for over 200 years. But we also became aware of the putrid smell and if Ilfracombe in January had seemed any more attractive we might have turned around there and then, abandoning our nth interview for a West Country general practice partnership. Fate being what it is we stayed, and got the job.

MALE MENOPAUSE

The Harris factory has now gone and the parking bay is double yellow lined. It was over a year after the factory had closed and seven years into my GP career that I provoked my mid-life crisis. I didn't 'decide' or 'resolve' to do research, I developed an obsession. GPs are supposed to be able to tolerate uncertainty – to have personalities that can repeatedly shrug off the fear that they have made a wrong decision. They are trained to press the bell and attack the next problem without lying awake at night. The fate of the Harris employees made redundant in 1982 was to cost me a lot of sleep.

I WONDER?

Some research is 'exploratory' – we need to know more about X and how Y and Z affect it. Other research is hypothesis-testing – 'I've a gut feeling that only Z affects X and I'm determined to prove it'. Riding hunches can certainly be exciting, even if it's not bareback, and can end in a painful fall. My first 'Harris hunch' was clear enough and selfishly motivated. The practice I had joined seemed extremely busy, busier than I liked. Much of the urgent demand ('I *must* see the doctor today') seemed to be Harris-generated. Slaughterers, pie-men, faggot-mixers, sausage-stuffers – and all the other players from the vegetarian's nightmare – had been brainwashed by the factory hygienists to consult us immediately about incipient or imaginary infections. Surely our practice workload should have dropped after the closure of the factory? Shouldn't our work stress have fallen as the life expectancy of Wiltshire pigs had risen? If I was able to prove that this phenomenon was real did it not have, by inverse extrapolation, implications for GP resource allocation? Should not practices still working in the hinterland of large industrial enterprises be better financed because of their extra workload? At least I had some experience of real research from my third year in Cambridge. I knew that I would need to read the relevant literature and put my ideas in the context of previous work. Actually there *was* no literature except for some poor-quality papers on the tangential subject of how enforced redundancy might affect the health of those losing their jobs. Suddenly I had a new and far less self-centred hunch. Dismounting is more graceful and less painful than being thrown and I changed to a new hypothesis – that the Harris ex-employees were going through a phase of deteriorating health consequent to their redundancy. Since most of them were registered at our practice I should be able to find, in their medical records, objective evidence to support my blueprint. I was no longer just obsessed, I was hypomanic.

DON'T SPECULATE, EXPERIMENT

John Hunter once said, famously, to his pupil Edward Jenner '… but why think, why not trie the Expt?'*. This is fine, but fieldwork takes time and effort. Our four-doctor practice in Calne was typical of contemporary UK general practice of that era in almost all respects except for the love–hate relationship with our high-cholesterol local industry. Partly out of shyness and partly out of realism ('no, you can't when we're so busy') I didn't discuss my research ambition with my partners for over a year. I gave up some of my own time (and that rightly belonging to my family) to travel to a Harris outpost in Ipswich to retrieve the personnel details of those who had been made redundant in Calne in July 1982. Intuition and dread

---

* Royal College of Surgeons of England (1976) *Letters from The Past: from John Hunter to Edward Jenner*. RCS, London. The letter quoted was dated 2 August, 1787.

of Hallam Street made me extract only names and addresses, but I think an ethics committee might have prevented me doing even this (I didn't realise that I needed permission). Back in Calne I began extracting, usually by night or over weekends, clinical data from the relevant medical records and expanded my 'participants' to households. I 'recruited', again by proxy, control families from other local industries that were still up and running. The index cards built up and the enthusiasm wilted as I began to look, more and more frantically, for the expected differences in consultation rates and so on, comparing before redundancy and after redundancy.

COMING OUT

It was just as well I was obsessed. It was at this time that I broke cover and was promptly told that I was wasting my time. This research was not exploratory, far too much of a gamble and, anyway, 'we don't need to know'. 'Unemployment is obviously bad for people, so obviously so that research is unnecessary' was the blunt opinion of one respected GP academic. On the other hand, the government in power in the mid-1980s (luxuriating in the lack of data) were asserting that the 3 million UK unemployed might be having some brief personal difficulties but that a streamlined economy would soon have them back into jobs that would be better and better paid. Against this backdrop there was no way that I could suggest to my partners that I have protected time away from my patients, but I did apply to the Scientific Foundation Board of our Royal College for a grant. Despite breaking the application protocols the SFB supported my work with a small grant (that was to be replenished twice, bless them) and I pressed on.

HELP!

By summer 1994 I was drowning in numbers and it was my wife who baled me out. Elaine would have had every justification in letting me go down with the ship but she seemed to know better than I did that I needed a statistician. A conversation across the coffee tray led to Susan Nethercott joining me at the index cards and within the space of two weekends she found statistically significant findings as expressed by the magic of p. In fact I had, by now, noticed a trend that suggested, graphically at least, that there was step up in GP workload from the time the Harris employees began to sense that their jobs might be 'on the line' and that the factory might close. We had discovered a phenomenon that is now well established – the adverse health implications of *insecure* employment. Susan was concerned by technical and highly mathematical anxieties that I couldn't hope to grasp and we sought the advice of Dr [now Professor] Ian Russell, a name that I had seen mentioned in *Pulse*. Ian was amazingly cooperative and I met him on Swindon station one windy evening. Over BR tea he whistled as he saw our findings. Then he pulled the pin and jumped on his train to Oxford. We were using the wrong statistical tests. We must go 'non-parametric' but … keep going! Susan rang him later in the week so that he could 'explain' and I could tell by her facial expression not only that she could understand but that she agreed.

JACKPOT

There are some people that one never forgets; likewise some names and phrases. One of mine is now 'the Mann–Whitney U Test'. The results were still highly significant and so was the phone call from Susan. The first paper we drafted was hopeless and didn't improve until we realised that we were writing at least three conclusions. In the end we published ten papers, eight in the *College Journal* (as it then was) and two in the *BMJ*. Unemployment was still a political 'hot potato' and the final insult to my family was when the media descended, scooped me up and made me famous for the requisite 15 minutes. After two days we dodged the leather-jacketed brigade camped on the lawn and fled – to the Lord Mayor's Show. For some reason we kept looking over our shoulders and not at the parade. Much more important to me was the MD degree that I obtained by writing a dissertation, donning a gown after 20 years and spending a sticky two hours with Lord Butterfield and three other professors.

POST MORTEM

I am still in full-time practice in Calne and I am still as boring as ever. At least Elaine doesn't have to look for the dreaded index cards under the car with a mirror before family holidays any more – the 'barnacle' days are over.* I now have the absolute pleasure of one full day per week of protected time for research which is funded by the R&D General Practice Scheme of my local NHSE. And I have just learned that our practice has been awarded a further three years support from the 'Culyer' fund. I can press on with my research into deprivation markers that might be appropriate for UK general practice. My hunch is … but never mind for now. Find your own! Even so I still have to be careful not to let all the fallout from being a 'research GP' impose on my leisure, on my family and on my practice. I now find myself writing chapters for books, advising others on the phone, refereeing papers for several journals, reviewing grant applications, speaking at 'away days' and fielding faxes from the Antipodes. 'See one, do one, teach one' seems to apply as much in the laboratory as at the bedside. But don't be put off. These days you can have your Weetabix before the battle. There are now Research and Development Support Units, Primary Care Research Networks, research clubs of all sorts, statisticians geared for advising in primary care, a host of individuals who have the teeshirt and the World Wide Web. You no longer have to pretend that 'I want to be alone'. There is no need.

* Desmond A and Moore J (1991) *Darwin*. Michael Joseph, London. Darwin's monograph on barnacles took 20 years to prepare and his children thought that all fathers spent their days studying molluscs!

15

University-based junior academic posts: overview and personal experiences

Crossing the Rubicon to Academus' garden?

Martin Underwood and Yvonne Carter

INTRODUCTION

Not only is more primary care-based research needed to strengthen the scientific foundations underpinning our work, but also the proportion of the undergraduate medical curriculum taught in primary care is increasing, probably up to 20% of clinical teaching within the next few years. Much of this research and teaching will be carried out by service general practitioners. These skills need developing during and after vocational training, both for those who will make this an important part of their future practice work and those who intend to pursue a full-time academic career. Compared to other medical specialities the number of academic GPs is small and their career structure is poorly developed. About 30% of the NHS's medical workforce are GPs, however, only 5–6% of academic posts are filled by GPs.[1]

A period of higher professional training for recent graduates of vocational training schemes (VTS) or extending vocational training to include academic training may benefit both future professors of general practice and future service GPs with research and teaching interests. The traditional career structure of general practice has made obtaining this difficult. However, the Primary Care Act[2] that permits the employment of salaried GPs, the availability of training awards (e.g. RCGP and MRC training fellowships) on a part-time basis and other pilot schemes suggest that opportunities for career flexibility are improving.

Further academic educational opportunities, either a longer period of vocational training or post-VTS salaried positions, are available at a number of medical schools. The London Initiative Zone Educational Incentives (LIZEI) scheme has provided extra financial resources to improve the educational opportunities in central London. Since 1995 it has made widely available, for the first time, post-VTS academic training offering a mixture of clinical work and higher professional training. All the London medical schools offer posts with different balance between clinical and educational activity, different educational activities and different degrees of involvement in their practices. At the time of writing it is not possible to predict which of these posts will continue after the end of LIZEI in 1998.

THE POSTS

It is beyond the scope of this chapter to review all of these posts. We will instead concentrate on four different models, provided at Queen Mary and Westfield College (QMW) (London Academic Training Scheme [LATS] Registrars, Academic Fellows, Academic Associates, Academic Trainees) and one at the University of Birmingham (Academic GP Registrar). They all have an emphasis on research training as the main educational activity and meet the training needs identified by the AUDGP.

These posts have a number of elements in common:

• developing a research project in any subject pertinent to general practice
• academic skills training
• personal supervision from a senior academic
• when appropriate, separate research or teaching supervision
• statistical and information technology support
• access to a mentor
• access to the other formal and informal educational activities that are part of the life of an academic department
• training for and participation in undergraduate teaching.

London Academic Training Scheme (LATS)

The LATS scheme is organised on a pan-London basis and funded directly from the NHS Executive. For the 1997/8 academic year, its third year of operation,

12 registrars were appointed, divided between the six London undergraduate schools and the University of Westminster. The appointments are for one year only. The registrars are full-time university employees whose time is split 70/30 between academic and clinical work. Their clinical work is in well-organised, usually training, practices where they have clinical duties only. The registrars attend the AUDGP's intensive three-day research methods course, based at St George's Medical School, at the start of the course and a weekly half-day educational session which provides ongoing formal training in research methods and an opportunity to meet the registrars from different schools.

Academic fellows

These posts are funded through the Education Boards of East London & the City and Redbridge & Waltham Forest Health Authorities. The appointments have been for up to 18 months, terminating at the end of LIZEI. Fellows are full-time university employees whose time is split 50/50 between academic and clinical work. Their clinical work is in developing practices where, in addition to clinical work, they spend time facilitating practice development. The time they spend in the practice releases the existing partners, either to participate in educational activities or to develop the practice.

Academic associates

These are funded through the Education Board of East London and the City Health Authority for up to 18 months, terminating at the end of LIZEI. They are GP principals who have joined a local practice that was having difficulty recruiting a new partner. They are part-time partners with all the consequent rights and responsibilities. In addition they are part-time employees of the university. They receive a pro rata share of practice profits plus a part-time university salary. At the end of the scheme it is expected that they will remain in their practices, possibly increasing their practice commitment. The split between the clinical and academic work varies but has always been at least half time in the practice.

Academic trainees

Academic trainees are not university employees. They are assistants who are employed by general practices. Their salary is reimbursed to the employing practice through a separate London Initiative Scheme programme, the 'Workforce Flexibility Scheme'. They are entitled to funding for educational activities under the LIZEI scheme. This funding pays for the time they spend on their academic work, plus a dowry to the academic department for the support they receive.

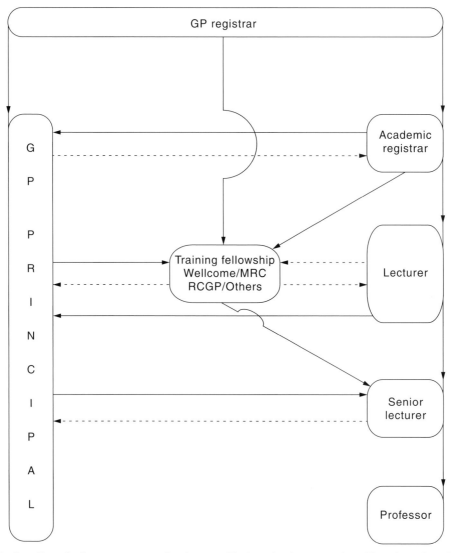

Broken lines indicate career paths that are likely to be less popular. The size of each box is not indicative of the number in that grade. There are other possible routes into and out of academic practice that are not marked on this figure.

Figure 15.1   Principal career paths into academic general practice

Academic GP registrars (Birmingham)

They are employed half time by the university as a lecturer, to develop a research proposal, and half time by a training practice as a GP registrar. Their GP registrar training is unchanged and during their university time they receive additional academic training. Funding is arranged from a variety of sources.

THE PARTICIPANTS

Most participants have developed their research ideas separate from ongoing departmental research. This avoids junior researchers joining an existing project simply to follow through someone else's original idea without fully developing their own critical faculties. However, the vertiginous early stages of the research learning curve and the long period between a new idea germinating and concrete results being obtained can be rather demoralising. This approach, although initially more challenging, is more likely to allow the participants to develop a lifetime of research interest and skills than the 'production line MD' required for higher training for many hospital specialities. An early indication of this has been the interest of several of the participants in pursuing MDs, based on their original ideas, after the end of their post. Increasing the number of MDs obtained by GPs from its historical low level (the RCGP was aware of 12 in 1995[3]) is an important part of developing a research culture in primary care.

Box 15.1   Some of the research topics tackled

- Management of oral anticoagulation in primary care
- GPs' attitudes to early discharge policies for patients with deliberate self-harm
- GPs' attitudes to antidepressant prescribing
- Folic acid awareness in Bengali and other pregnant women
- Improving uptake of mammography in inner London
- Ethnic differences in the use of hormone replacement therapy
- Sensitivity and specificity of GPs' diagnoses of asthma
- Iron deficiency anaemia in Bengali children
- Quality of undergraduate teaching

HOW DO THESE POSTS FIT INTO THE STRUCTURE OF ACADEMIC TRAINING?

Plans are being developed to make working towards a research-based Masters degree an integral part of any future LATS or similar posts. These will then fit firmly into the first level of progression through training for academic general practice, with the next steps being completion of an MSc and starting work on either an MD or a PhD. Because the amount of clinical work in these posts, particularly the LATS posts, is comparatively low, they could be seen as sinecures by colleagues in full-time service general practice. Evidence of achievement towards acquiring a Masters degree will help to counter this perception.

It is, however, important that in the pursuit of academic honours junior academic trainees do not neglect the need to win their spurs as clinicians. If they do not gain sufficient grass roots' clinical experience they will not have the practical knowledge base from which to develop their research and teaching. This may affect their credibility when called on to act as leaders of the profession later in their careers.

Many may wish to sample life in an academic department but not all will want to pursue an academic career, although three-quarters of those who become academics would make the same career choice again.[4] Even if they do not want to cross the Rubicon to Academus' garden, either immediately or later in their careers they will enrich general practice overall. At the very least they might learn not to mix Roman and Greek metaphors.

Consumers' experience of academic training

Johanna Cornwell

Since completing vocational training I have been a LATS registrar and subsequently an Academic Fellow in the Department of General Practice and Primary Care at QMW. These posts are provided for young general practitioners who, after vocational training, want to defer going into a partnership. They provide an opportunity to develop research and teaching skills while continuing clinical practice.

BECOMING A MEMBER OF A DEPARTMENT

Part of the enjoyment of the schemes is becoming a member of a department of general practice and learning about academic general practice in an experiential manner. It is important for the registrars or fellows to feel welcomed and integrated into the department. In a large department this can be problematic.

Being in a department offers the opportunity to gain first-hand experience of an academic GP's work, including juggling clinical, research and teaching activities. Learning to prioritise is an important skill for a junior academic to develop. The pressure of applying for ethical approval and funding, and the highs or lows (depending on the outcome) associated with this are fundamental to an academic career. The unpleasant experience of completed research being rejected for publication can be demoralising; determination and persistence are required.

Attendance at the local and annual AUDGP scientific meetings is an excellent opportunity to meet colleagues from different departments, to hear about different research areas and to present your own work.

RESEARCH

LATS registrars spend 70% of their time on research and teaching, including a weekly half-day release course, hosted by a different department each term, allowing interaction with senior academics with a wide range of interests. Formal seminars focus on research methods, critical appraisal, presentation skills and, in the final term, a group project. A variety of expert speakers facilitate the sessions. Most subjects are dictated by the expressed needs of the group. The registrars are encouraged to formulate and present their own research ideas to the group in the first term, with updates through the year and a more formal presentation at the end of the year. This is useful preparation for presenting research at conferences.

Informal sessions, similar to VTS half-day release, are held on alternate weeks. Clinical problems, any departmental difficulties and future career plans are also aired. These sessions are facilitated by one senior lecturer experienced in group work, providing continuity and supporting development of a group identity.

The remaining academic time is devoted to projects based in the registrar's host department. There is considerable flexibility in the projects the registrars undertake. A notable achievement of the scheme is the encouragement to pursue an original research idea of interest.

At the beginning of the year registrars are encouraged to keep a journal of their experiences and thoughts. It was a useful exercise and, although not religiously adhered to, it is instructive as a tool to witness personal development through the scheme. Reflecting on it now, it is interesting to read about the time taken to get the project up and running, the disheartening periods when the research wasn't going according to plan and the buzz when it was going well with interesting results.

Academic Fellows devote half their time to academic work, developing their own research ideas; one session of this is spent attending the departmental academic skills course with a focus on research methods and presenting research ideas for critical appraisal. Practical subjects such as information technology and presentation skills were included. Although these posts are longer than the one-year LATS posts, they are more pressured because of the larger clinical commitment.

SUPERVISION

High-quality project supervision by the host department is the key to success of the posts. This provision varied between departments and in my department was partly determined by the registrars'/fellows' research interests.

Project supervisors provide regular supervision and help to formulate an idea into an answerable hypothesis, then give guidance on appropriate methodology. Practical skills acquired included collecting and handling data, an introduction to computer statistics packages and appropriate statistical tests, and writing up the study with consideration of how the research is to be disseminated, including publication and presentation at conferences.

Both the registrars and fellows require a lot of support when first starting, particularly to identify a practical research question. For the one-year LATS posts this is particularly important.

The registrars/fellows are supervised by a senior lecturer, with regular meetings on an individual basis to discuss research, its progress and future plans. One of the priorities in this time was considering undertaking a higher degree and the work that this would entail.

Choosing a research supervisor

Points to consider:

- Can a good working relationship be established?
- Is he or she willing and able to set aside the time to provide regular supervision?
- Does he or she have a special interest/knowledge of chosen research area?

MENTORS

Dependent on individual need, a personal mentor is available. If required, mentors can help with research, clinical or emotional problems. The mentors come from a variety of clinical and non-clinical backgrounds.

TEACHING

Both schemes encourage participation in undergraduate teaching. Commitment to this is flexible; some LATS registrars concentrate on undergraduate teaching and a related project rather than pure research. Teaching opportunities include supervising assignment projects for fourth-year medical students, and teaching communication and clinical skills to first-year clinical students. Training courses are available. Although an enjoyable and rewarding aspect of the posts, teaching can reduce the time available for research.

CLINICAL ATTACHMENT

The clinical commitment for LATS registrars is three sessions, for one year. One partner acts as their clinical mentor and will discuss clinical problems as necessary. For the apprehensive registrar who has just completed vocational training this is a supportive environment; independence is encouraged but help and advice are available if needed.

The clinical commitment for Academic Fellows is five sessions, and they are attached to a small practice to assist in practice development. The fellows have some choice in their placement, and are able to select the practice from a shortlist. At the beginning of the post they are encouraged by their supervisor to consider carefully the distribution of clinical sessions through the week, taking account of academic commitments. This facilitates negotiation with the practice about use of time at the surgery. The fellow provides the principal with the time to undertake practice and/or personal development.

One session is specifically allocated to practice development. Areas targeted by the fellows include updating the practice computer, computerising repeat prescribing and developing protocols. Because the fellows are not partners and do not have a say in the practices' decision-making processes, implementation can be difficult. Furthermore, what might seem an appropriate area by the fellow could have cost or workload implications for the practice.

THE FUTURE

After completing the scheme the registrars/fellows are equipped with the knowledge and skills to make a more informed decision about their future careers. Future plans may include entering a full-time partnership, combined clinical and academic general practice or a change of career, e.g. to public health medicine. Those who want an academic career will have acquired many of the requisite skills and work for a higher degree may be well underway.

Box 15.2   Good aspects of the scheme

- The opportunity to try something new
- Encouraged diversity and flexibility
- Time to think and read about research and develop own ideas
- Good grounding in research methods
- Access to supervision and expert advice
- Hands-on experience of the heartache of doing research
- Experience of applying for ethical approval and funding
- Writing up a research project for presentation and publication
- Learning teaching and presentation skills
- Encouragement to pursue a higher degree

Box 15.3   Ways in which the scheme could be improved

- Availability of longer appointments to facilitate completion of research
- Opportunity to undertake a taught Masters degree

David Fitzmaurice

INTRODUCTION

I was appointed as the first academic GP registrar at Birmingham University in October 1992. This was a two-year post consisting of five sessions as a lecturer and five sessions as a GP registrar. I had broad commitments within the department, the balance of the post favouring research over teaching. I planned to establish a research project suitable for submission for a higher degree by the end of two years; this was partially achieved.

PHYSICAL OUTCOME

My initial research interest was comparing the use of different inhalers for asthma, which I planned to develop into an MD proposal. I made more progress researching into management of anticoagulation in general practice, and this is now the basis of my proposed MD.

My main teaching commitment has been in a communication skills course for postgraduate training, which developed from an interest in communication across the primary/secondary care interface[5] into being principal tutor on communication skills courses. With support from a senior lecturer in communication skills I produced new training material, supervised training of role players, supervised undergraduate and postgraduate training courses and developed training packages for external use.

I had a half-time GP registrar commitment in an inner-city practice with 7000 patients, with close links to the university and another full-time GP registrar. Being both a registrar and a lecturer led to an assumption that my training needs were different to other registrars. Although lecturers have more 'protected time' for reading, it was still difficult to have enough time for personal learning. The supervisors within the department of general practice were aware of this, and allowed withdrawal from other departmental commitments to make up for it.

To fulfil training requirements, it is necessary to attend a VTS course for one year, either half time for two years or full time for one year. I chose the latter but lost contact with my VTS peers before I could sit MRCGP towards the end of my second year.

While my training was equivalent to that received by full-time registrars, there are difficulties for trainers in the organisation of tutorials for people learning at different rates. If the academic registrar posts are to flourish it is important that training needs are not overlooked. Academic registrars need a normal registrar's relationship with their practice and trainer.

GP registrars are usually considered to have different workloads from GP principals.[6–8] More recently this has been questioned.[9] I had approximately 75% of the patient contact of a full-time registrar in the practice for new patient contacts, follow-up patients and 'extra' patients, and 50% for 'out-of-hours' work. Time can be wasted travelling between practice and department. Allowance needs to be made for the geographical separation, the sessions spent in the practice and the registrar's need to experience the fluctuations in the practice week.

Psychological outcome

Prioritising service and academic activities is a problem for academic GPs. Since GP registrar posts are supernumerary, this was not a major problem. My academic work had positive benefits on my enthusiasm for clinical work. It can be difficult to be fully involved in an academic department when employed part time.[10] However, few members of the department work full time and I felt 'involved' in departmental decision making, although as the most junior clinical member of the department one's opinions carry little weight.

Adjusting from a hospital SHO post to learning and teaching general practice was difficult. The problems all registrars experience were present: home visits, geographical disorientation, identifying the roles and identities of the primary healthcare team. Additionally there were problems because colleagues' expectations could be different compared to those of other registrars. These problems were minimised by attending the Central Birmingham VTS scheme for the whole of my two years of hospital-based vocational training. Switching between the registrar and lecturer roles was at times quite difficult.

Intellectually, the lecturer experience, with protected time for research essential for the success of any research post, allowed me to rediscover the questioning attitudes which originally attracted me to medicine.

As a relatively recent graduate it was exciting to be able to influence, even in a small way, the stultifying nature of undergraduate medical education. My main input was as a facilitator for GP tutors who do most of the formal undergraduate general practice teaching. I was a conduit between the department of general practice and the tutors, allowing a free flow of ideas between the main parties involved in undergraduate training.

SOCIAL OUTCOME

The reduced contact with other registrars and being part time made my life more difficult. I missed the valuable mutual support available through VTS groups in my second year. Being a registrar representative to the Midland Faculty of the RCGP partially addressed this; however, formal feedback to other registrars was difficult. Attendance at regional study days allowed some contact, although there could be problems for registrars who are new to a region.

One major consideration for anyone thinking about an academic career is finance. It was difficult financially, changing from a hospital job as a fourth-year SHO. A lecturer's salary is £3000 less than a GP registrar's. By taking an academic option my salary drop was larger than that experienced by most registrars – my salary fell by £7500. This could be a problem for doctors who have financial commitments based on previous earnings. I did additional locum work to supplement my income. This can interfere with clinical performance and personal development. Efforts at a political level are needed both to obtain income equity between GP registrars and hospital trainees and to address the longer-term earnings loss for academic GPs.[11]

When appointed I was concerned that being part time I would be marginalised within the practice.[10] However, I became increasingly involved in the practice, spending more time in the practice than my sessional commitment. Working half time over two years may allow registrars to acquire a greater insight into practice affairs than a one-year post. The academic element encourages an enthusiastic approach to clinical work, that may protect against burn-out in later life.

DISCUSSION

General practice needs a stronger academic base to provide the research and teaching base for a sustainable primary care-led NHS. Until recently almost all medical undergraduate teaching was based on hospital practice and there is not yet a widespread culture of research in primary care. To promote and encourage the expansion of academic general practice a career structure is needed that enables younger doctors to consider this option.[12]

Overall, I think my post has been successful, with a definite improvement in my morale and enthusiasm for medicine. This might have occurred simply as a result of leaving hospital medicine. However, the sum of GP training with protected time for academic training has been greater than its parts. Time management is vitally important and the weekly timetable needs careful thought. The training needs of the academic registrar must not be underestimated. There were many positive aspects to this post; however, the financial penalty for entering academia is substantial. This may deter talented candidates from applying.

CONCLUSION

My experience as a GP registrar and lecturer allowed the development of research and teaching skills within a university department with a wide range of resources. My GP training and clinical experience has been comparable to full-time GP registrars, and the two-year, half-time option may allow a greater insight into general practice than the traditional registrar year. There are problems but, apart from the income drop, they are relatively minor. I can thoroughly recommend it.

REFERENCES

1. Medical Research Council (1997) *MRC Topic Review, Primary Health Care 1997*. Medical Research Council, London.

2. National Health Service (Primary Care) Act 1997 (commencement No. 3) Order 1997.

3. *RCGP Members' Reference Book 1996* (1996) Royal College of General Practitioners, London.

4. Richards R (1997) *Clinical Academic Careers: report of independent task force*. CVCP, London.

5. Prasher V, Fitzmaurice D, Krishnan VHR and Oyebode F (1992) Communication between general practitioners and psychiatrists. *Psychiatric Bulletin*. **16**: 468–9.

6. Stubbings CA and Gowers JI (1979) A comparison of trainee and trainer clinical experience. *Journal of the Royal College of General Practitioners*. **29**: 47–52.

7. Carney TA (1979) Clinical experience of a trainee in general practice. *Journal of the Royal College of General Practitioners.* **29**: 40–4.

8. Hasler JC (1983) Do trainees see patients with chronic illness? *BMJ.* **287**: 1679–82.

9. Eccles M, Bamford C, Steen N and Russell I (1994) Casemix and content of trainee consultations: findings from the north of England study of standards and performance in general practice. *British Journal of General Practitioners.* **44**: 437–40.

10. Handysides S (1994) A career structure for general practice. *BMJ.* **308**: 253–6.

11. Mant D (1997) *R&D in Primary Care National Working Party Report.* Department of Health, London.

12. Association of University Departments of General Practice (1993) A career structure for academic general practice. Leicester AUDGP Conference.

16

Health services research

in general practice:

an inner city perspective

Chris Griffiths and Gene Feder

INTRODUCTION

The growing importance of health services research

Health services research tackles questions about the provision of healthcare to individuals and populations, using a range of methodologies. Its importance has grown in the past 20 years as healthcare demands have outstripped resources in all healthcare systems, and large variations in the volume and quality of care have become apparent even with national systems. Health services research traditionally has focused on secondary and tertiary care, partly because of the concentration of resources in these services and partly because of the greater availability of routinely collected patient and process of care data. As the centre of gravity within the NHS moves towards primary care and chronic disease management shifts towards medical and nursing care into the community, research on the appropriateness and effectiveness of general practice is essential.

In this chapter we describe personal perspectives and experiences gained from seven years of health services research in East London. During this period we have carried out studies on different clinical topics adapting methods from various disciplines. We have picked four of these studies to illustrate some of the lessons we have learned on the way. Our account will show how concrete research questions emerge from specific contexts, how the question and the context lead to a particular study design, the obstacles which invariably arise from trying to apply a research protocol and how the results lead to further research questions.

East London as a setting for health services research: problems and opportunities

East London comprises three of the most deprived boroughs in the UK: Hackney, Newham and Tower Hamlets. Furthermore, census data suggest that levels of deprivation have increased further in the last ten years.[1] East London has traditionally been a port of first call for many refugee communities, initially reflecting its proximity to the Port of London, more recently the fact that local accommodation is relatively cheap. In addition to the settled Jewish, Bengali and Afro-Caribbean communities, the last decade has seen influxes of Turkish, Kurdish and Somali groups; the most recent arrivals have been families from the former Yugoslavia and those displaced from volcanic eruptions in Montserrat.

General practitioners in the area provide high levels of care in the face of enormous difficulties. Poor surgery premises, a highly mobile population with practice list turnovers of 25–30% per year, differences in first language spoken by doctor and patient combine to make general practice a demanding occupation.[1] The variety of resident populations is mirrored in the styles of general practice. The area has a high proportion of single-handed practitioners (many without practice nursing or manager support), but also has a number of large well-developed group practices. Most practitioners have little time in which to take part in research, although there is now a growing network of university-linked practices and a new primary care research network.

Against this background we have often envied those carrying out health services research in areas more conducive to research, where populations are stable and served by a single hospital, and where most patients have telephones and most dutifully complete questionnaires without reminders. On the other hand, it is the nature of health services research that many questions emerging from general practice in East London or other large urban areas cannot be answered by studies based in Oxford or Hampshire. East London is an area of great richness and variety and there are many opportunities for research. The creativity of local communities in the face of severe socioeconomic pressures and the striving of many general practices to meet the demands of their patients creates exciting challenges for researchers.

Four studies

We have chosen four studies comprising two randomised trials, an ecological analysis of asthma morbidity and a study testing the feasibility of a new technology (portable spirometers) in primary care. Brief summaries of these are given below:

- **Study A: Do clinical guidelines introduced with practice-based education improve care of asthmatic and diabetic patients?**[2] In 1994, we completed a randomised trial testing the effect of local asthma and diabetes guidelines dissemination to non-training practices in Hackney. Twenty four practices were recruited and randomised to two groups; each group received one of the two guidelines through practice-based educational visits, while providing data for both conditions. Process measures for the two conditions assessed one year later showed significant improvements in all diabetes quality of care measures and two of seven asthma measures. The trial served as a model for the subsequent guidelines programme in East London, was widely cited and was one of the first health services research papers abstracted in the journal *Evidence-based Medicine.*
- **Study B: Do guidelines-derived postal prompts to survivors of myocardial infarction or unstable angina and to their GPs improve secondary prevention?**[3] Moving to the enhancement of guidelines implementation, this ongoing randomised trial tests the effect on uptake of (pharmacological and lifestyle) secondary prevention measures of sending postal prompts to patients discharged after a coronary event and to their GPs. The study therefore tests the potential of involving patients in behaviour change as a way of implementing guidelines. The main outcome measures are rates of cholesterol testing, lipid-lowering drug and beta-blocker prescribing. Fifty eight of 60 Hackney practices agreed to take part (only two declined) and were randomised to receive prompts or usual care. We have completed patient recruitment and are in the final stages of data collection. Alongside this trial we carried out a parallel qualitative study investigating the acceptability of the intervention to patients and GPs.[4]
- **Study C: Admissions for asthma in East London: associations with characteristics of local general practices, prescribing and population.**[5] Hospital admission rates for asthma in East London are among the highest in the UK. Admission rates vary between practices. This ecological study attempted to determine which general practice, prescribing and population factors were most strongly associated with high asthma admission rates among all 163 practices in East London and the City Health Authority. Colleagues had previously validated the use of the practice asthma prophylaxis to bronchodilator ratio as a marker of appropriate asthma prescribing in these practices. This study looked at the relative importance of prescribing in relation to other factors that could influence hospital admission. We found that single-handed practice was the factor most strongly related to high admission rates.

- **Study D: Can spirometry be used in primary care to help identify and manage patients with chronic obstructive airways disease? Interim results from a study in East London.**[6] As a response to the recommendation in the nascent British Thoracic Society's chronic obstructive pulmonary disease (COPD) guidelines that spirometry should be the gold standard test of lung function when considering a diagnosis of COPD, we are testing the feasibility of spirometry carried out by specialist respiratory nurses in three group practices. We invited all patients aged 50 years and over listed on the practices' asthma registers to sessions testing reversibility to bronchodilator and, if appropriate, response to a steroid trial.

CHOOSING A RESEARCH QUESTION (AND OUR FIRST 'LAW' OF HEALTH SERVICES RESEARCH)

In each of these studies, the underlying question was a response to local circumstances and national changes in the organisation of healthcare. Our first law of health services research is that the need for research and its complexity is proportional to the rate of organisational change in health services. This is good news for those looking for an open-ended supply of research topics, but – in the continual re-engineering of the NHS – bad for those seeking a quiet life.

Testing methods of guidelines dissemination and implementation

The expectation of commissioners and (some) clinicians that guidelines could work as tools for quality improvement, together with the relative paucity of research on their efficacy made guidelines a topic crying out for research. Our first trial was a response to the purchaser provider split precipitated by the 1989 Government NHS White Paper, which led to a request to our department to develop primary care guidelines, including referral recommendations. Before embarking on guidelines development we searched for evidence that they could influence primary care. We were disappointed: few studies had been carried out in the UK. Our realisation that no one knew how to make guidelines work in general practice led us to combine development of local guidelines with study (A).

Our second trial (B) followed naturally from the first, testing the possibility of involving patients directly in guidelines implementation through postal prompts. From the first trial we knew that guidelines could make a positive difference in practice and felt compelled to investigate how this effect could be enhanced. Our enthusiasm for exploring this issue further was reinforced by research on guidelines becoming fashionable and a favoured topic for support from the NHS R&D programme.

Primary care factors that affect asthma admission rates; an analysis crossing the primary–secondary care interface

The search for valid markers of prescribing quality, again a response to health services development[7] was a prelude to our ecological study addressing variations in asthma admission rates by local practice. The East London general practice research database has details of all local practices, including resourcing (e.g. nursing support), prescribing (e.g. PACT data), activity (e.g. cervical cytology uptake) and population data (from census reports) and has proved a powerful research tool in a number of areas.[8] We had already shown a significant univariate relationship between practice asthma prescribing and their asthma admission rates; practices with higher ratios of asthma prophylaxis to bronchodilator ratios tended to have fewer patients admitted to hospitals. Our research question followed directly from that finding: is this association outweighed by other factors such as the deprivation of the practice population or the style of practice? That high admission rates represented a local healthcare issue of some importance meant the study was able to address a fascinating area of unexplained variations in care.

Testing a new technology in general practice

The development of new COPD guidelines with largely untested recommendations for use of spirometry provided an opportunity to assess the feasibility of a new diagnostic method in primary care. The emphasis on asthma management over the last decade has meant that diagnostic distinctions between COPD and asthma have received little attention. While we could have addressed issues such as sensitivity and specificity of the diagnostic method, a more relevant question was the rate of potential misdiagnosis, i.e. what proportion of patients on practice asthma registers had lung function consistent with a diagnosis of COPD? Asthma registers in East London were growing in size and we were concerned that the (justifiable) low threshold for using prophylactic anti-inflammatory (steroid) therapy for asthma patients may have led to overprescribing of steroids routinely in patients with COPD.

CHOOSING A STUDY DESIGN (AND OUR SECOND LAW OF HEALTH SERVICES RESEARCH)

The basic designs of the four studies followed logically from the questions we were trying to answer. However, our second law of health services research – and probably all research – is that the study design is a compromise between what you would like to achieve and what is feasible in practice.

The Hawthorne effect

The challenge in our first study (A) was to test the efficacy of a guidelines dissemination strategy. While the most powerful design was clearly a randomised trial, we faced the question of whether we should include a control group in which practices received no support. There were two strong arguments against this. First, we soon recognised that non-training practices, many of which had no particular interest in research, would be unlikely to take part if we approached them offering a 50:50 chance of being randomised to a control arm where they would receive nothing, save having researchers trawl through their records and publish the results. Second, a control group without any involvement in the research left us vulnerable to the Hawthorne effect when interpreting the effect of the intervention. The Hawthorne effect can be described as the change in behaviour of a system (in this case, general practices) resulting from involvement in a research study.

We were fortunate that an early discussion with a trial methodologist revealed this pitfall, which crops up repeatedly in health services research. Evaluations of guidelines programmes often could not disentangle improvements in care from the increased attention of having an intervention from the specific effect of introducing a guideline. We therefore chose a balanced incomplete block design, whereby each group of practices receives a different guideline, but provides data for both conditions, in this case asthma and diabetes. This illustrates an important point: discussion of trial design with an experienced methodologist is a good use of time in the planning stage. We have also found close early and continuing collaboration with a statistician essential for the quality of our quantitative studies.

In our second trial (B) we chose not to use a balanced incomplete block design for two reasons: first, our credibility among practices which had developed from the first trial and other work in East London meant we were more confident of a high rate of practice recruitment; second, our intervention was much more low key (postal information only), reducing the potential size of a Hawthorne effect. The only difference between our contact with intervention and control practices was the intervention itself.

Factorial designs

The intervention in the second (B) trial had two components: postal information to patients and to GPs. One possibility was to use a factorial design of four groups of practices: no intervention, postal prompts to patients, postal prompts to GPs and postal prompts to both patients and GPs. This design would satisfy purists who want to know the separate effect of the two aspects of the intervention. We compromised by having two groups (no postal prompts versus prompts to both GP and patient) because the factorial design would have required more practices to achieve the same statistical power and because we reasoned that the cost of sending information to both GP and patient in the real world was minimal. The distinction between the two elements of the intervention would have been truly academic.

What's in the black box? The place of qualitative studies alongside pragmatic health service research trials

Health services research trials often test an intervention made up of multiple components – a 'black box'. If such an intervention is effective it is difficult to know why it was acceptable to patients or clinicians or how its effect could be enhanced. One approach that we have used has been to carry out a qualitative study in parallel with a randomised trial, with the aim of finding out in detail how the intervention affects (or fails to affect) participants within the trial. This raises its own difficulties; in particular, interviewing participants in a trial may alter their behaviour and compromise the study.

In the case of our second trial (B), we chose to interview patients about their response to postal prompts and will analyse our trial data with these patients included and excluded. Interviewing GPs participating in the study about their response to the intervention would have fatally biased our trial (there were many fewer practices than patients in the trial); we reached a compromise by exposing a selection of GPs from the next borough to the intervention and then asking their views. Another benefit of carrying out a parallel qualitative study is that it can help in predicting whether an intervention is likely to work in another setting, for instance, a suburban, rather than an inner city area, increasing the generalisability of the findings.

The use of routinely available data

Our ecological study of asthma admission rates is notable for using data which have been gathered originally for purposes other than research. Thus, asthma admissions data are routinely collected for the Hospital In-patient Enquiry, prescribing data are collected by PACT (Prescribing Analysis and CosT), socioeconomic data on populations are part of the ten-yearly census, and practice characteristics are routinely collected by health authorities. A study is considerably cheaper if these types of data can be used. One important disadvantage is that the available data may not be exactly what you require for your study. For example, numbers of claims for payment for night visits done by practices are available, but actual numbers of visits made are not: thus a poorly organised practice may underclaim and hence visits will be underestimated. A second disadvantage is that it is difficult to check accuracy of routinely collected data retrospectively. A third disadvantage of non-health service routinely collected data is that they may not be directly attributable to patients. Socioeconomic status from the census can only be crudely mapped on to practice data at ward level and vice versa.

The use of disease registers as a sampling frame

Study A and our study of COPD diagnosis (D) required us to sample practice asthma registers. Research that makes use of practices' disease registers as a means of identifying patients for a study faces a particular difficulty. In an ideal world, all practices would have identical diagnostic criteria for a given condition; these would be applied in the same way between practices, and all practices would have equally efficient administrative mechanisms for adding patients to registers and removing them when they move from the practice, develop inactive disease or die. The reality is that practices use registers in individual and idiosyncratic ways. In our study of the feasibility of spirometry, we sampled disease registers for asthma from three practices. Two used their registers to give *point* prevalence of asthma (i.e. patients could be 'inactivated' on registers) and the other practice's register represented a *cumulative* prevalence of asthma. Thus the use of disease registers represents a compromise. However, the possible alternatives of screening the practice population or attempting to validate the diagnosis from the notes is time-consuming and often impractical. Moreover, if patient identification is part of the intervention, using disease registers – despite their heterogeneity – means that the intervention can be used in routine practice (i.e. it is a pragmatic method rather than a pure research tool).

CARRYING THROUGH RESEARCH DESIGNS (AND OUR THIRD LAW OF HEALTH SERVICES RESEARCH)

Practice recruitment

Health services research interventions are often at the level of the practice, rather than the individual patient. Thus testing efficacy through a randomised design will require randomisation of practices, rather than patients. Recruiting adequate numbers requires researchers to have effective strategies for practice recruitment. Hence our third law of health services research: you cannot be too careful in approaching practices for participation in studies (and it helps if you are perceived as a colleague rather than an 'alien' researcher).

Although a practice's main criterion will be time commitment in studies, there are several ways of maximising chances of recruitment. Murphy *et al.*[9] have articulated an approach, which we have adapted to good effect for our studies. Key strategies are: writing a relatively brief letter to practices describing the study and then following up the letter with a telephone call a week later. This call is not to ask for a definitive response, but to clarify and give more information. Targeting this call to the person who has the relevant responsibility for the decision saves time. An offer of a visit to discuss the work may help at this point but it is our experience that practices will often agree to take part at this point, provided the study does not involve them in too much administrative or clinical work. We think the largely positive response from practices stems from the identification of fellow East London GPs among the research team, a choice of topics compatible with GP's own priorities and a consistent attempt to minimise the time commitment of the practice to the study.

Keeping a study running on time

Randomised trials involving large numbers of practices may involve a programme of rolling recruitment and hence rolling intervention. Data may need to be collected at tightly controlled time points. In these situations it is easy for schedules to slip, particularly when data are collected from patients directly, for instance, by interview. Two strategies that can help are first, to set up a study steering group with overall responsibility. A second is to set up electronic reminder systems within the study database that prompt timely data collection or even print appropriate letters.

Process measures, intermediate outcomes and outcome measures

Outcomes that matter for patients and the health service – death, disability and hospitalisation – are relatively rare even in high-risk groups. Therefore studies which use these to assess the effect of an intervention are too large for a local study. Therefore, in health services and clinical research it is often necessary to use process measures signifying quality of care (e.g. appropriate prescribing) or intermediate outcomes (e.g. patient symptoms). In trial A the partly validated steroid:bronchodilator prescribing ratio and in trial B, aspirin and statin prescribing were used as measures, relying on other research which links these to 'true' outcomes. In study D, respiratory symptom scores (and spirometry) were intermediate outcome measures.

FURTHER RESEARCH QUESTIONS (AND THE FOURTH LAW OF HEALTH SERVICES RESEARCH)

Guidelines studies

Our first trial of guidelines dissemination led to a second study in which we tested the effects of involving patients themselves in guidelines implementation. Many questions about guidelines implementation remain: how can we implement more than one guideline at a time? Are nurse educators as effective as doctors in changing practice? How can we prolong the effect of an intervention?

Studies of factors influencing asthma admission rates

Although our study of asthma admission rates included sociodemographic data, practice characteristics and practice prescribing, several questions remain. What effect would possible confounders such as pollution and variations in local asthma prevalence have on our results? Was our finding of an association between high practice asthma admission rates and single-handed practice a phenomenon of deprived inner city areas? We intend to address these through a study which includes not only East London, but also the neighbouring Barking and Havering, so bringing into the analysis less deprived areas. This study will also include data on traffic flows (as a marker of pollution) and surveys of asthma prevalence.

Research questions arising from spirometric assessment of patients on asthma registers

Several questions arose from this piece of work. First, we found that at least a third of patients had good lung function (FEV1 >75% predicted). Did these patients have well controlled asthma or were they patients who have never justified a diagnosis of asthma? Second, do COPD patients who are not responsive to a steroid trial need to continue inhaled steroids? Trials addressing this issue are due to report in the near future. Anecdotally, we noticed that some of our patients in this category who stopped inhaled steroids subsequently suffered exacerbations of COPD and were restarted on inhaled steroids. Is this justified? Can inhaled steroids reduce the rate of exacerbations in these patients even though they have little or no objective lung function response to a two week course of oral steroids?

Our fourth law of research is obvious: as soon as you answer one question, many spring up to replace it. Genuine questions are not the problem, time and money are!

CONCLUSION

This chapter has illustrated some of the decisions and opportunities that faced us during the course of four research studies in East London. Perhaps the most important point this account illustrates is the welter of potential questions and methodologies which face the primary health services researcher. Pragmatism and opportunism are essential requirements for this type of research. Focusing on answerable, locally relevant but generalisable questions makes health services in primary care feasible and rewarding.

REFERENCES

1. ELCHA (1996) Health in the East End, annual public health report *1995–6*. East London and the City Health Authority, London.

2. Feder G, Griffiths C, Highton C, Spence M, Eldridge S and Southgate L (1995) Do clinical guidelines introduced with practice-based education improve care of asthmatic and diabetic patients? *BMJ.* **311**: 1473–8.

3. Feder G, Griffiths C, Spence M and Eldridge S (1996) Do guidelines-derived postal prompts to survivors of myocardial infarction or unstable angina and to their GPs improve secondary prevention? *Family Practice.* **13**(3): 346.

4. Feder G, Griffiths C, Hillier S and Formby J (1997) *After the Infarct Report: views of east London patients, GPs and practice nurses. Final Report.* Dept of General Practice and Primary Care, St Bartholomew's and The Royal London School of Medicine and Dentistry, London.

5. Griffiths C, Sturdy P, Naish J, Omar R, Dolan S and Feder G (1997) Admissions for asthma in east London: associations with characteristics of local general practices, prescribing and population. *BMJ.* **314**: 482–6.

6. Griffiths C, Foster G, Feder G, Wedzicha J and Marlow G (1998) Can spirometry be used in primary care to help identify and manage patients with chronic obstructive pulmonary disease? Interim results from a study in East London. Association of University Departments of General Practice. Annual Scientific Meeting (Abstract).

7. Jones I (1994) *Prescription for Improvement.* Audit Commission, HMSO, London.

8. Griffiths C, Naish J, Sturdy P and Pereira F (1996) *Prescribing and hospital admissions for asthma in east London.* BMJ. **312**: 481–2.

9. Murphy E, Spiegal N and Kinmonth AL (1992) Will you help me with my research? Gaining access to primary care settings and subjects. *British Journal of General Practice.* **42**(357): 162–5.

17

Nursing research

in primary care

Fiona Ross

INTRODUCTION

This chapter discusses present trends and activities in nursing research in primary care, drawing on insights from history, literature and personal experience. The first section identifies the political and professional context in which research takes place in primary care and the position of nursing within it. Issues such as research training, funding opportunities, and the implications for nursing of policies supporting evidence-based practice and cross-professional boundary work are addressed. Margaret Elliot puts the flesh on the bones with her description of the experience of undertaking research training and completing a practice-based study while engaged in a busy clinical role.

Nursing in primary healthcare covers a wide range of activities embracing generalists and specialists. This heterogeneity is reflected in the different origins, roles, activities, structures and power relationships within the nursing system. The work is invisible, the patient/client groups are often at the margins, or displaced, and the work may be episodic, long-term and incorporate social as well as family care. The generalist in primary care, seeks to understand and treat the whole individual within an established and continuing relationship. Thus the challenge for research in this field is enormous.

Research in nursing is young, diverse and eclectic in terms of its underpinning disciplines and the focus. In many ways it is similar to research in general practice, which is also an emerging discipline struggling for respectability and credibility within an arena dominated by bioscience and clinical research.

Early beginnings of research in primary care nursing

The questions that policy makers were asking about community nursing 30 years ago were not so different from concerns expressed today. The optimum deployment of skills in the community nursing workforce was the focus of important research undertaken by Lisbeth Hockey at the Queen's Nursing Institute in London. A nurse and a graduate of the London School of Economics, Hockey used diary records and questionnaires as data collection methods for workload analysis of district nursing terms.[1-4] Four key studies, undertaken in the late 1960s and early 1970s, represent a rare example of a programme of work in community nursing, with funding provided by a charitable organisation. It is a reflection of short-termism that this type of programme funding is scarce in nursing research today.

Another important and early contribution was the work of Charlotte Kratz.[5] Using a qualitative method, which was unusual at the time, she studied the care of patients recovering from stroke at home and developed a 'continuum of care' theory. This identified appropriate focused care for the acutely ill and inappropriate, diffuse care for those patients who were getting better, but still had dependency needs. Kratz also introduced the concepts of 'managing' and 'fairness'. She argued that district nurses justify their minimal care of the chronic sick in terms of the patient and his or her family's obligation to manage. If these patients express extra demands for care, above those defined by the nurse, it is perceived as unfair, because it inevitably deprives others of nursing time. Again this work is seminal, because of the innovative, qualitative method and for the development of an analytical framework outlining district nursing priorities for intervention. It is interesting to note that these early and important contributions to community nursing research were made by women who were important professional leaders and opinion formers within nursing, academia and journalism.

Current issues

From these early beginnings there has been further progress. Baker *et al.*[6] conducted a review of community nursing research. They identified that of the empirical studies published between 1974 and 1982, the majority concerned health visiting, one third addressed district nursing and the investigators/principal authors were dominated by the medical profession.

Rafferty and Traynor[7] describe research as a 'game with sponsors, players, structure, rules and organisation ... a team sport ... it has stars and spectators, requires long years of training, coaching and an extended apprenticeship. Finally and above all else it is thought to thrive on competition'. With these characteristics in mind, how can we measure and monitor the performance of research in nursing and what criteria can we use to characterise the quality of the research culture? In other words, how does nursing research in primary care measure up in this game? Mulhall[8] argues that the low status of nursing and thereby its research is manifest in its funding problems. The strategy for research[9] notes that overall, the investment in nursing research is small and success in securing funding from the research councils is infinitesimal. With the late entry of nursing into higher education it is comparatively rare for nurses to pursue a full-time research career, which means there are few role models, mentors and an acute shortage of nurses available to supervise higher degrees. These problems are amplified in the less 'glamorous' sectors in nursing, for example care of the elderly and primary care.

The new Centre for Policy and Nursing Research, based at the London School of Hygiene and Tropical Medicine aims to map the activity and distribution of nursing research.[9] The early findings from this work indicate that PhD output more than doubled between 1978 and 1992; not surprisingly the universities with the highest outputs are ones where there has been the longest tradition of academic nursing, for example Manchester and Edinburgh. The main source of funding was from the health service, with only 1% coming from the research councils.[10] The popular topics were education, service organisation and workforce. In contrast the least popular topic was related to patient experience and satisfaction. However, the proportion of these PhDs carried out by nurses researching questions generated by primary care is not clear.

RESEARCH DEVELOPMENT IN PRIMARY CARE NURSING

Although there is growth in doctorally prepared nurses it would seem that it is still the exception for these individuals to develop a research career in programme leadership. The first chair in community nursing was funded by the Queen's Nursing Institute at Manchester University in the late 1980s. Throughout the 1990s there has been a growth in established chairs in community nursing at King's College London, Liverpool, Glasgow Caledonian and Hull. These developments have made a difference to the fragmented nature of community nursing research and have enabled the development of emergent programmes and research training in the field. The following is only a selection from recent developments to indicate the development of research themes in these settings:

- decision making in district nursing, needs assessment and care management (Jean McIntosh, Glasgow Caledonian University)
- patient/consumer perspectives, professional and practice development at the primary/secondary care interface (Sally Kendall, Centre for Research in Primary Health Care at Buckinghamshire University College)

- needs assessment and the evaluation of care provision matched with identified needs (Alison While and Sarah Cowley, King's College London).

Policy directives to move towards a primary care-led NHS, evidence-based practice and knowledgeable practitioners present a mountain of challenges for research. Peeling off the layers of the rhetoric, we are left with the reality of a diminishing and ageing workforce of district nurses and health visitors.[11] In the last seven years there has been a fourfold increase in numbers of practice nurses working in a mixture of delegated and autonomous roles undertaking a range of tasks and activities for which they are variously trained. Therefore within primary care there is a dynamic tension between professional boundaries as medical substitution and independent practice evolves, providing fertile ground for many research questions, for example:

- demand versus needs-led service
- individual versus population approaches
- generalists versus specialists
- professional interests versus organisational priorities
- diversity versus standardisation.

Some examples of current work investigating aspects of some of the above issues are:

- the cultural differences between nursing and medicine using an ethnographic approach (Anne Williams and a team at the National Primary Care Research and Development Centre, Manchester)
- the impact of fundholding on district nursing using a case study method (Claire Goodman at the University of Hertfordshire)
- the evaluation of different models of integrated nursing teams in three health authorities (Fiona Ross and Pit Rink at St George's Hospital Medical School, London).

Carrying out the work and managing grants and projects is only one part of the 'game' alluded to by Rafferty and Traynor. Increasingly, nurses are becoming players in policy development and priority setting at the centre. Nurses with academic backgrounds in primary care have been members of the Central Committee for Research and Development, notably Karen Luker and Deborah Hennessy. Influencing shifts in thinking at policy-making level will come about slowly as nurses develop research credibility.

FUTURE PRIORITIES

There are many ways of cutting the cake to identify future research priorities. A recent topic review in primary healthcare carried out by the Medical Research Council[12] identified the following as important areas for investigation:

- health/help-seeking behaviour

- social and healthcare boundary
- treatment and care pathways
- workforce roles, substitution and skill mix
- new roles in nursing e.g. care management.

Over the last ten years there has been a move towards qualitative methods in nursing. The debate on the 'quantitative/qualitative divide' has become rather sterile. It is important that the strengths of both approaches and the way in which they can be utilised to answer particular research questions are recognised.[13] For example, the use of inductive methods to develop theoretical underpinning for interventions and to explore the context and meaning of illness in primary care is increasingly advocated.[12] Nurse researchers are gaining considerable experience in qualitative methods, which is possibly an untapped resource, but could enhance the development of interdisciplinary research teams.

The national framework for R&D within the NHS was laid down in 1991[9] and emphasised the importance of capacity-building and developing career structures in research. Nursing has a long way to go in this regard. The opportunities for research training studentships and fellowships are limited. Recognising this as a problem, the MRC has earmarked two clinical training fellowships for professions allied to medicine (PAMS). Regional fellowships offer another route which offer equivalent salary for 3 years to enable research training and doctoral study in a university setting. Studentships are also available through the MRC, but none of these to date have been secured by a general practitioner so the likelihood of nurses succeeding is poor. These limited opportunities for full-time, fully funded research training mean that often nurses do part-time PhDs on top of work and domestic responsibilities. The time-frame to completion is long, and the impetus to publish and the motivation to continue is often exhausted in the process.

As well as the shortage of opportunities for research training, with some exceptions, there is a scarcity of nurse leaders to carry out research in primary care. There is not a tradition within nursing to carry out post-doctoral work in order to gain project management and supervisory skills. Nurses gaining doctorates tend to get swallowed up in education or health service management, which results in fragmented rather than programme research. Systemic problems with marginalisation from decision making and limited opportunities for funding are not unique to nursing, but are also experienced by other groups such as social scientists and PAMS in health services research where the biomedical sciences and empiricism are powerful.

MOVING FORWARD

Evidence-based practice, although not a new idea in nursing, offers the potential for change. In the 1970s, Briggs[14] exhorted nursing to be research based and this has been a common theme in numerous policy documents since. The implementation of evidence-based practice through the use of clinical guidelines is contested territory. It has been argued that it is a mechanism of imposing external control within a healthcare system that is inherently uncertain,[15] especially where the only acceptable level of evidence is that generated from the randomised control trial (RCT). As Kendall[16] notes, there are dangers in limiting research approaches to the RCT, which denies the rich diversity of human experience that nurses working in the community have the privilege to be intimate with.

Identifying ways in which research can be implemented is currently a priority for the NHS. There are many approaches, but in South Thames we are running a large project funded by the Regional Office, which aims to evaluate the effectiveness of practice development roles in implementing evidence-based clinical guidelines into nine clinical settings using change management (STEP project). This project is not only a collaboration between academic departments of nursing in South Thames, the practice development posts have been established, funded and will function under joint management arrangements between the university and a partner trust. Four of these projects are being carried out in primary care.

The future presents opportunities as well as threats. On the one hand we need to preserve a system where it is possible to conduct work that seeks to develop nursing theory so that nursing research can play a full and informed part in the multidisciplinary research of the health services agenda. However, we also need to consider other strategies that allow research to be embedded in practice and to avoid past criticisms that nursing research is elitist. McGloughlin,[17] in a provocative editorial, challenges nursing research to play a key role in the NHS R&D agenda: 'it must take stock of the real position of the profession in the R&D stakes rather than the aspirational one which is reflected through the professional rhetoric'.

The direction of funding and R&D policy is determined by the needs of the health service and effectiveness. These issues are wider than nursing alone and require staff with a range of research skills and from different disciplines. The enriching and developmental process of working with other disciplines is not easy and there may be tensions over intellectual property, conflict relating to leadership, attribution of outputs for the research assessment exercise and the often delicate matter of authorship order on publications.

Working together means the difficult, intellectual and often emotionally demanding task of listening carefully to the unfamiliar scientific territory of researchers from different backgrounds and working to integrate these ideas in the design, analysis and reporting of studies. This means taking risks, trusting, having clearly defined roles and agreement on roles, responsibilities, ownership of ideas and authorship of papers. Interprofessional research and methodological pluralism can benefit nurse-led research, but we need to choose our partners wisely, be confident and vigilant.

Nursing in primary care has a developing intellectual culture that needs nurturing. Rafferty and Traynor argue that we need to build that capital as quickly as possible by creating teams with a broad spectrum of skills and expertise.[10] Nurse-led health services research needs to work with other disciplines, such as social sciences and health economics, and move away from the rather insular grooming of nurse researchers. We need to keep in mind how the research we do will make a difference to patients and to the service and from this, work out the best way to get there.

PERSONAL REFLECTIONS

Most researchers in nursing probably can point to the lucky break in their careers that opened up the job or put them in contact with the mentor, who gave support and encouragement. This is probably not unique to nursing, but reflects a professional structure which lacks established career structures in research. As an undergraduate I was influenced by eminent nurse academics such as Annie Altshcul and Lisbeth Hockey, who urged that nurses should always ask questions and work to systematically analyse practice. After some time as a district nurse I was fortunate to engineer a joint appointment district nurse/research in a London Department of General Practice (St Thomas' Hospital with Professor David Morrell). As well as maintaining a clinical role I was able to participate in and learn about research in primary care as well as undertaking my own PhD study. Following this I worked in academic roles in a Department of Nursing Studies (King's College London) and as a post-doctoral senior lecturer in the Department of General Practice (St George's Hospital Medical School). The latter was the first senior academic appointment for a nurse in a Medical School, Department of General Practice. This gave me invaluable experience working across disciplinary boundaries in research and teaching. In the last five years there has been a growth in such posts across the UK, which bodes well for building the interdisciplinary research teams of the future in primary care.

REFERENCES

1. Hockey L (1966) *Feeling the Pulse: a survey of district nursing in six areas.* Queen's Institute of District Nursing, London.

2. Hockey L (1968) *Care in the Balance: a study of collaboration between hospital and community services.* Queen's Institute of District Nursing, London.

3. Hockey L and Buttimore A (1970) *Co-operation in Patient Care.* Queen's Institute of District Nursing, London.

4. Hockey L (1972) *Use or Abuse? A study of the state enrolled nurse in the local authority nursing services.* Queen's Institute of District Nursing, London.

5. Kratz C (1978) *Care of the Long Term Sick in the Community.* Churchill Livingstone, Edinburgh.

6. Baker G, Bevan J, McDonnell L and Wall B (1987) *Community Nursing Research and Recent Developments.* Croom Helm, London.

7. Rafferty AM and Traynor M (1997) On the state of play in nursing research. *Journal of Interprofessional Care.* **11**(1): 43–8.

8. Mulhall A (1995) Nursing research: what difference does it make? *Journal of Advanced Nursing.* **21**: 576–83.

9. DoH (1991) *Research for Health: a research and development strategy for the NHS.* HMSO, London.

10. Rafferty AM and Traynor M (1997) Quality and quantity in research policy for nursing. *Nursing Times Research.* **2**(1): 16–27.

11. Audit Commission (1997) *Wards without Walls: a study of the efficiency and effectiveness of community nursing services.* Consultative document. Audit Commission, London.

12. Medical Research Council (1997) *Primary Health Care: topic review.* MRC, London.

13. Black N (1996) Why we need observational studies to evaluate the effectiveness of health care. *BMJ.* **312**: 1215–18.

14. Briggs A (1972) *Report of the Committee on Nursing.* Cmnd 5115. HMSO, London.

15. Dean K and Hunter D (1996) New directions for health: towards a knowledge base for public health action. *Social Science and Medicine.* **42**(5): 745–50.

16. Kendall S (1997) What do we mean by evidence? Implications for primary health care nursing. *Journal of Interprofessional Care.* **11**(1): 23–35.

17. McGloughlin C (1996) Purchasing R&D in nursing: its role in the shared agenda to improve the NHS. *Nursing Times Research.* **1**(6): 409–11.

Nursing research in primary care

Margaret Elliott

INTRODUCTION

Two years ago, I completed a research project in primary healthcare which, at the time, I believed was the end of a stimulating mental journey. Since then I have discovered that it was just the beginning. Hopefully, in this chapter I can relate some of the opportunities and difficulties that I encountered while undertaking the project and also impart some of my enthusiasm for the research process.

THE FIRST STEPS

In 1984, when I became a registered general nurse, conducting research or having a degree were not important issues for me or for the nursing environment in which I worked. In 1990, I moved into a management post in a community trust as a team leader of district nurses and health visitors. At that time, a few managers had management degrees and some nurses were undertaking post-registration degrees in community nursing. I became aware that to enhance my career prospects within the NHS and more importantly for my own self-esteem, I needed a degree-level qualification, which implicitly meant undertaking research. Enabling this idea to become a reality required perseverance, with minimal support or advice from managers. The two main problems that arose were: identifying an appropriate course; and paying the course fees. As few of the nurse managers had academic qualifications, they did not always see the important connection between research training and the nurse's role.

I regularly scanned the nursing press for a suitable course and eventually saw a two-year, part-time MSc course in health sciences. I had no knowledge of the level of study that an MSc would require and did not know anyone at work who could advise me on the appropriateness of the course or my ability to complete it. I had not studied for a number of years, had read very little research and had no experience of conducting research. But I did have an understanding of management principles, experience of quality assurance, a good command of English and, significantly, a strong desire to gain graduate status and to increase my understanding of research, so I decided to apply. Coincidentally, I had seen a notice calling for 'applications for course funding' from the regional health authority. I applied for funding, the RHA approved and my manager agreed to give me one day off a week. The research content of the course included research and statistics modules, and a research dissertation. I embarked on this course of study with limited experience of undertaking literature searches, using libraries or computers, no comprehension of statistics and little knowledge of research methodologies – I was on a sharp but fascinating learning curve.

THE RESEARCH PROJECT

The policy background to my study was the NHS and Community Care Act[1] and the concomitant issues of: measuring and evaluating quality of care; identifying local health needs; working in partnership with clients and professionals; and the separation of health and social care. In reality, some care can be undertaken by both or either services and this can lead to duplications or omissions in service provision if planning is not effectively coordinated. In the community trust where my research took place, clients with health and social needs received both district nursing and home care services and the services were managed and budgeted separately.

Considering the issues mentioned above, it was thought appropriate to collect baseline data with the aim of describing clients over 65 years old who used both services. The objectives were to measure their functional status, to compare their levels of satisfaction with both services, and to identify omissions and duplications in service provision. This was a small, descriptive, quantitative study utilising five 'assessment-of-functional-status' questionnaires, a client-satisfaction questionnaire,[2] professional interviews and a record audit. Fifteen clients and 17 professionals were interviewed. The results showed that the clients were elderly – between 80 and 99 years old – and functionally dependent. Over 50% had probable depression, but the professionals focused on physical rather than psychosocial needs. The district nursing service scored generally higher satisfaction scores, but both services had low scores for client participation in care and a theme of dissatisfaction with the allocation of time emerged. The majority of professionals reported poor communication and a lack of liaison between the services, and duplications in service provision were occurring.

Overview of the process

The aim of the research process at first or second degree level is not to produce 'researchers', but to equip health professionals with critical appraisal skills and with an understanding of the research process (*see* Box 17.1). This process is

---

Box 17.1   The research process

- Finding a supervisor
- Undertaking a literature search
- Reviewing the literature
- Writing a proposal
- Gaining approval from the local ethics committee
- Reviewing further literature
- Conducting the research
- Analysing the results
- Writing the report
- Post-research benefits

complex and without previous experience it can appear daunting. It has also been said that if anything can go wrong then it probably will. I found that to reduce any potential problems, conducting research requires self-discipline, supportive family, friends and work colleagues, perseverance and the ability to use or develop project management skills. For example, divide the whole operation into short, manageable pieces of work; methodically plan; negotiate; devise an overall time plan; study regularly; and establish how you work most effectively.

Finding a supervisor

Finding or being allocated a supervisor who has experience or an interest in your field of study is very important. Being part of a taught course usually means that students are allocated supervisors. Throughout the research process I met with my supervisor every two months to discuss my progress and any potential or actual problems. The meetings were essential to provide deadlines to complete pieces of work and to motivate me to continue. Having a supportive supervisor was significant in guiding and developing me as a researcher, enhancing the experience and making the project enjoyable and stimulating.

Undertaking a literature search

The ability to conduct a literature search is central to the research process. Usually, searches are conducted in a university library with the aid of computer technology. Some libraries provide regular teaching sessions, and this was my introduction to finding my way around the wealth of material available. I consulted the literature at two stages of the process: before writing the proposal, to assist in defining the topic; and before conducting the research, to provide material for theoretical and methodological frameworks,[3] and to be able to compare my results with previously reported studies. Before starting the literature search, I found it helpful to brainstorm key topics and words connected with the project, forming links between the words to produce groups of topics. These topic groups then became the main headings for the literature search. For example, my study's topic groups were: community policies; care management; interprofessional collaboration; community services; and evaluation of quality. I spent hours in the library; once I had started searching I became obsessed with the task, culminating in photocopying reams of articles.

Reviewing the literature

Reviewing and evaluating the relevant literature is fundamental to conducting research. The first stage of review (before writing the proposal) can be conducted quite quickly because it forms only a short section of the proposal. However, the second stage of review (before conducting the research), is a time-consuming task; it requires systematic frameworks for coherent analysis and synthesis. It was at this point that I began to allot myself regular study periods. My most effective method of working was to allocate four hours of uninterrupted time: reading and classifying articles requires concentration and methodical note taking. I separated articles into their topic headings, highlighted relevant sentences, summarised pertinent subtopics from each article on 'post-it' stickers, and then typed sentences under their subject headings into the computer. It seems to me that it is better to start writing incoherent paragraphs than not to start writing at all.

Writing the proposal

At first, writing the proposal seemed a daunting task even with advice from my supervisor on the proposal design. I felt that, at this early stage in the process, I did not fully understand the whole operation, plus I had never written a formal proposal before. The actual production of a proposal is very logical, helped by the availability of structured frameworks to follow. In retrospect, my difficulties in this area arose from two problems: having to please several 'masters'; and the theory–practice gap. As my study time was funded by my workplace, the nursing management insisted on influencing the proposal methodology. On the one hand, I had to satisfy my supervisor that the proposal was academically robust and that I would be able to complete it within six months. On the other hand, I needed approval for the proposal from the directors of the district nursing and home care services to grant me access to the sites. Perseverance, planning and negotiation skills were required to keep everyone happy.

The second difficulty arose as a consequence of the theory–practice gap. Part of the essential learning connected with any subject includes understanding the related language and terms. The taught modules of the course and further reading provided me with the theory; however, I was not sure of the full significance of some of the terminology and concepts. These did not become clear until the end of the research process when I could reflect on the practical aspects of the operation. Despite these problems, I found this period to be the beginning of a mentally stimulating, creative experience.

The local ethics committee

Gaining ethical approval for research is essential for the protection of potential subjects, but with poor project-planning, ethical approval can be viewed as a barrier. Ethics committees sit regularly, but with varying frequency. You need to find out the local meeting dates and prepare the proposal with enough time before the project start date to send the paper to the committee, or to present it in person, which some committees require. I found that making contact with the committee secretary enabled me to gather helpful information, particularly when I was asked to attend to present my proposal. This procedure caused me some apprehension, but I now consider it to have been a valuable learning experience. There also needs to be enough time to make any suggested modifications to the proposal that the committee might request before granting approval. Taking heed of these planning points will reduce anxiety enormously.

Reviewing further literature

Comments on this section are provided under the headings of 'undertaking a literature search' and 'reviewing the literature'.

Conducting the research

Conducting the research was the most interesting part of the process, because finally I was actually collecting the data. From this period onwards the project became so absorbing that it often became detrimental to my work commitments. My project utilised a multi-method approach: five 'assessment-of-functional-status' questionnaires; a client-satisfaction questionnaire; professional interviews; and record audit. This produced rich data for the study, provided me with a greater awareness of when and how to use different research methods, and increased my confidence and skill in interview techniques. On reflection, I found being an 'in-house' researcher advantageous, as access to staff and patients was easy and the study was relevant to my clinical and managerial role.

Analysing the results

All data need interpretation using statistical analyses and presentation. This section of the study was the most challenging, because I had never used a statistics package before and was nervous about applying statistical analyses correctly. For the same reasons, it was also the most rewarding because I succeeded in a new and difficult area. I used a freeware, statistics package called Epi. Info, and initially sought help to use the program from the university epidemiological department. I did not attempt complex statistical techniques, but employed simple methods, such as producing means, medians, standard deviations and correlation. Presentation of the data became more creative through computer technology: for example bar charts, graphs, contrasting colours, highlighting and different fonts were some of the options I used.

Writing the report

The study is not complete until the report is written and disseminated, but writing requires discipline. There is a standard framework for writing research reports which must be followed and which provides a logical reflection of the whole process and a known format for critical appraisal. I had taken the practical advice that when studying you need a designated study area; but I had not followed the advice of writing up sections of the report as they are completed to avoid frantic activity at the end of the project.[4] To compound this frantic state, although the deadline for handing in the report was imminent, cleaning the house seemed a far more important task; procrastination is easy, but self-discipline is essential. As time was running out, this part of the study became the most stressful. This is when my family and work colleagues needed to be at their most supportive. I had to take time off work, miss lectures at university and ignore my social life to complete the report. Fortunately, being part of a taught course meant that everyone was experiencing the same feelings at the same time, which was reassuring.

Post-research benefits

After I had finished the report I felt euphoric; I had put a huge amount of effort into this piece of work and finally I had achieved my goal and had a social life again. However, at the back of my mind was the acknowledgement that research should be widely disseminated, and this meant writing an article for publication. I wanted to write an article, but needed some time away from the research. It was a year before I had both the time and inclination to write again.

Following completion of this project I have experienced many positive outcomes at home and work, which are interlinked. I gained valuable practice in the art of writing, in computer skills, research techniques and the research process. Because of this I have learnt to be more analytical, critical and logical in my thought processes. This has resulted in work colleagues asking for my opinions on issues and I have the confidence to give constructive, critical feedback. This in turn has raised my self-esteem, which is reflected both at work and at home. I have since been motivated to undertake further research and have made two applications for research fellowship funding and an application to the NHSE, all of which have been rejected. It is difficult to find funding for nursing research. I have also felt inspired and able to write several articles which have been published. I have made connections with other professionals who I would not normally have met, which has opened up further work possibilities. I feel less daunted by the idea of taking on different or extra work, because I have faith in my abilities to plan, conduct and write a good piece of work.

REFERENCES

1. Department of Health (1990) *National Health Service and Community Care Act.* HMSO, London.

2. Elliot M (1997) Health and social care in the community. *Elderly Care.* **9**(2): 22–6.

3. Cormack DFS (ed) (1991) *The Research Process in Nursing*, 2nd edn. Blackwell Scientific Publications, Oxford.

4. Bell J (1993) *Doing Your Research Project. A guide for first-time researchers in education and social science*, 2nd edn. Open University Press, Buckingham.

18

The interface between pharmacy and primary care

Geoffrey Harding and Kevin Taylor

The pharmacists' place in primary care

INTRODUCTION

There are approximately 12 000 community pharmacies in Great Britain, typified by the high-street chemist. They comprise independent shops (owned and managed by individuals), small chains, large multiples (for instance Boots the Chemists) and, increasingly, in-store pharmacies within supermarkets.

In the past, pharmacists' activities centred around the manufacture of medicines from their constituent ingredients and their supply in accordance with physicians' prescriptions. However, the rapid expansion of the pharmaceutical industry in the latter half of the 20th century has all but abolished the need for pharmacists to compound medicines. This, together with the advent of original pack dispensing, where packs of medication are produced by industry with information inserts for direct supply to patients, and with the proliferation of computer technology in pharmacies and general practitioners' surgeries, has forced a reappraisal of pharmacists' activities. In response to an independent review of pharmacy by the Nuffield Foundation[1] and subsequent government White Papers, pharmacists have sought to redefine their role and have extended their activities beyond dispensing prescribed medication. Thus, increasingly, pharmacists are providing healthcare advice to the public and other health workers, treating minor ailments and performing some minor diagnostic testing.

The primary healthcare team

In discussions of primary healthcare and the primary healthcare team, pharmacy is frequently either omitted or considered to be very much at the periphery. This may reflect the physical separation of pharmacists from other health workers and/or the ambiguous nature of pharmacy's status, as both a professional and commercial activity. Indeed this 'role strain' or role ambiguity, resulting from the apparently conflicting demands of commercialism and professionalism, has been the focus of much published research on pharmacists' activities.

Changing roles in healthcare

Recent NHS reforms in pursuit of cost-effective health services, for instance nurse prescribing and reclassification of medicines formerly only available with a prescription as Pharmacy Medicines and now openly available from pharmacies, have resulted in the blurring of the traditional boundaries of professional responsibility. The distinct possibility that pharmacists will in the future be given authority to diagnose conditions such as asthma and dispense items such as antibiotics without a prescription indicates that professional boundaries will continue to be redrawn.

Such developments may not initially be welcomed by all health workers – perceiving this as 'boundary encroachment' as one profession apparently 'poaches' ground previously outside its territory. Nevertheless, successful provision of health services to the public requires communication, cooperation and collaboration between members of the primary healthcare team. However, the dynamics of the relationships between team members are poorly characterised and the relationships with pharmacists particularly so.

Evaluation of primary care pharmacy research in the UK

The historical development of pharmacy-based research has been patchy, and most early research concentrated on the role and function of hospital pharmacists. The inauguration of the College of Pharmacy Practice in 1981 promoted research into primary care pharmacy research. The introduction of the Department of Health-sponsored Pharmacy Practice Research Enterprise Scheme in 1990 and the formation of Pharmacy Practice Research Resource Centre and establishment of the *International Journal of Pharmacy Practice* in 1991 have consolidated the position of primary care pharmacy research in both academia and the health service.

An extensive independent review of published UK health services research in pharmacy, which included primary care pharmacy research, was conducted by Mays in 1994.[2] This found that:

- most research had been conducted in a hospital setting
- most studies were descriptive and the data not fully exploited
- there were few evaluative studies and they were often of 'dubious quality'
- data were often collected by pharmacists providing the service or intervention being studied and this was uncontrolled for bias
- studies were often carried out in isolation from other health services researchers
- the pursuit of research by pharmacists alone had resulted in pharmacist-driven research that risked lack of rigour and objectivity
- few practice researchers had adopted a truly multidisciplinary approach to service evaluation or attempted to adopt existing evaluative research designs.

PHARMACIST–GP INTERACTIONS

A number of factors may inhibit effective cooperation between health professionals, such as differences in status, prestige and power of the individual team members. Additionally, inadequate communication and poor appreciation of each others' roles may hinder the development of a more team-based approach to healthcare.

Although pharmacists may liaise with a number of members of the primary healthcare team, including district nurses and dentists, they most frequently interact with general medical practitioners. A fully developed relationship between pharmacists and general practitioners would appear to be particularly mutually beneficial. Pharmacists' knowledge base encompasses all aspects of medicines' use. Their knowledge of therapeutic indications, costs, suitable alternatives, etc. could be of considerable benefit to GPs under pressure to prescribe cost-effectively, while the diagnosis and treatment of minor illness relieves the burden of patient numbers for GPs and offers pharmacies opportunities to enhance their profitability through appropriate sales of medicines.

A POSSIBLE RESEARCH AGENDA FOR INTERPROFESSIONAL RELATIONS IN PRIMARY CARE PHARMACY

Very little is known about the interprofessional relationship between pharmacists and GPs. For example, does physical proximity influence collaboration and exchange of expertise? Indeed Mays' review of research into pharmacy practice[2] specifically highlighted that studies of interprofessional relationships formed one of the principal gaps in current UK primary care pharmacy research. A possible research agenda within this field might include:

- What role can pharmacists play in reducing the demand on GPs' time?
- Do pharmacists have a role in the supply of repeat prescriptions?
- Are the activities of GPs, practice nurses and pharmacists complementary or duplicating?
- How cost-effective is the pharmacist's role?
- How might interprofessional communication be enhanced?

PUBLISHED RESEARCH INTO PHARMACIST– GP RELATIONS

A number of studies have attempted to ascertain GPs' opinions about pharmacists extending their activities. These suggest that pharmacists and GPs are broadly in agreement about pharmacists' current input into prescribing, but that GPs are more reticent about pharmacists' involvement in more innovative developments, such as providing screening services and keeping patient medication records.[3,4] One study reported that GPs had positive attitudes towards pharmacists involvement in advising patients about minor illness, identifying adverse drug reactions and advising GPs about cost-effective prescribing.[5] These GPs were, however, divided about pharmacists providing screening services, supervising repeat prescribing or monitoring medicines in residential homes. Negative attitudes have been expressed by GPs towards pharmacists advising patients about adverse drug reactions, unless the patient is referred back to their GP,[6] and many GPs believe that the commercial nature of pharmacists' work leads to bias in their health promotion activities.

Communication and collaboration between GPs and pharmacists has been poorly characterised. It is generally informal and is limited by the physical separation of GPs' surgeries and pharmacies. Indeed, pharmacists are legally required to be constantly present in the pharmacy to supervise dispensing and the sale of

Pharmacy Medicines. It has also been suggested that a psychological barrier to closer working may result from pharmacists 'normally' only contacting GPs to query a prescription, which may be interpreted by GPs as a challenge to their professional authority.[1] The Royal Commission on the NHS in 1979, encouraged the development of health centres having integral pharmacies, as a means of promoting pharmacists' integration within the healthcare team. Our own work has suggested that when pharmacists and GPs are brought together within the environment of a health centre, interprofessional communication and collaboration is enhanced compared to the traditional arrangement.[6] However, notwithstanding GPs' positive perception of them, pharmacists, even in health centres, perceived their role to be passive and supportive to the GP.

CURRENT STATUS OF PRIMARY CARE RESEARCH IN PHARMACY

In Britain, primary care pharmacy has been a long-neglected area of research. The majority of research has been published in the last decade – generally under the heading of pharmacy practice research. Pharmacy practice research has been defined as:[7]

> ... research which attempts to understand pharmacy and the way in which it is practised, in order to support the objectives of pharmacy practice and to ensure that pharmacists' knowledge and skills are used to best effect in solving the problems of the health service and meeting the needs of the population. (p. 8)

Much of this research has developed from concerns about what pharmacists do during the course of their work. Thus it has comprised primarily an audit of pharmacists' activities (which reflects the ongoing debate within pharmacy regarding its role and function in the late 20th century), while the broader issue of pharmacists' integrated role and function within a primary healthcare team has received relatively little attention. Because of its embryonic nature, research in primary care pharmacy is, perhaps not surprisingly, characterised by isolation from other disciplines, based on limited funding and has had little impact on policy. A major stumbling block in this respect is the fact that the commercial environment in which primary care pharmacy is practised needs to be adequately addressed. Indeed, it is the largely unique blend of private and public service provision delivered from a state subsidised business that offers a particularly innovative research agenda.

RESEARCH RESOURCES FOR PRIMARY CARE PHARMACY RESEARCH

Research networks

To consolidate the research base of primary care pharmacy, research networks have been established nationwide. Some are highly structured, while others are little more than a loose confederation of individuals interested in conducting research. Research networks serve as a useful starting point for novice researchers. Networks provide an infrastructure for:

- multi-site research
- large-scale data collection
- support in both research and development.

Funding

Funding for primary care pharmacy projects generally derives from one of three sources:

- Commissioned research: this funding is for research which is overtly policy-related, with the research question predefined (occasionally with predefined methodologies) by the funding body. Such bodies include: the Department of Health, Welsh Office and Scottish Home and Health Department, The Royal Pharmaceutical Society of Great Britain and local health authorities.
- Responsive funding: these are grants awarded in open competition by a number of bodies on the basis of proposals submitted by researchers. They incorporate a range of schemes, from small grants for sundry expenses such as stationery, administrative support, etc. to large grants for research programmes lasting years and covering salary and institutional costs. Grant-awarding institutions for primary care pharmacy research include Economic and Social Research Council, Medical Research Council, Department of Health, NHS Research and Development, Galen and Linstead awards (both administered by the Royal Pharmaceutical Society), charitable trusts such as Nuffield Trust, Wellcome Institute, Royal College of General Practitioners and the European Union.
- *Ad hoc*/commercial funding sources: in the context of primary care pharmacy research funding might be sought from pharmaceutical companies.

Resources for information and advice on methodology and statistical analysis

- Web sites: there are a number of web sites located on the Internet which are dedicated to pharmacy. Most notable of these is Pharm Web (http://pharmweb1.man). This web site contains a considerable volume of information of direct relevance to primary care pharmacy, and includes sections of publications, a calendar of forthcoming conferences and meetings, courses and teaching information and discussion groups.
- Pharmacy Practice Research Resource Centre, Department of Pharmacy, University of Manchester, Manchester M13 9PL (0161 275 2415/2342) provides a range of support services to researchers, including literature searches, etc.
- Academic practice units based in hospitals, although serving as a link between academic and hospital pharmacy, are a potential resource for primary care pharmacy research.
- Royal Pharmaceutical Society of Great Britain, 1 Lambeth High Street, London SE1 4JN (0171 735 9141), the governing body of pharmacy in the UK, has a library holding an extensive collection of specialist journals.
- A number of university departments, including general practice, primary care and public health, may offer some form of consultancy support service to primary care practitioners. Additionally, there are pharmacy related departments in the following institutions:
  - Derby: Pharmacy Academic Practice Unit, University of Derby, School of Health and Community Studies, Chevin Avenue, Mickleover, Derby DE3 5GX (01332 622222)
  - Keele: Department of Pharmacy Policy and Practice, Keele University, Keele, Staffordshire ST5 5BG (01782 583444)
  - Leeds: Division of Academic Pharmacy Practice, University of Leeds, Leeds LS2 9NS (0113 283 3113).
- Computer abstraction services. In addition to Medline, the Bath Information Data Services (BIDS) incorporates a range of databases of which ISI Citation indexes are particularly useful for research in primary care pharmacy.
- UK Schools of Pharmacy. Primary care pharmacy research is actively undertaken in these institutions:
  - Aberdeen: School of Pharmacy, Robert Gordon University, Schoolhill, Aberdeen AB9 1FR (01224 262520)
  - Bath: School of Pharmacy and Pharmacology, University of Bath, Claverton Down, Bath BA2 7AY (01225 826789)
  - Belfast: School of Pharmacy, Medical Biology Centre, The Queen's University of Belfast, 97 Lisburn Road, Belfast BT9 7BL (01232 245133)
  - Birmingham: Department of Pharmaceutical and Biological Sciences, Aston University, Aston Triangle, Birmingham B4 7ET (0121 359 3611)

- Bradford: School of Pharmacy, University of Bradford, Bradford, West Yorkshire BD7 1DP (01274 384661)
- Brighton: Department of Pharmacy, University of Brighton, Lewes Road, Brighton BN2 4GJ (01273 642074)
- Cardiff: Welsh School of Pharmacy, University of Wales College Cardiff, King Edward VII Avenue, Cardiff CF1 3XF (01222 874080)
- Leicester: Department of Pharmaceutical Sciences, De Montfort University, The Gateway, Leicester LE1 9BH (0116 257 7270)
- Liverpool: School of Pharmacy and Chemistry, Liverpool John Moores University, Byrom Street, Liverpool L3 3AF (0151 231 2097)
- London: Department of Pharmacy, King's College London, Manresa Road, London SW3 6LX (0171 333 4787); School of Pharmacy, University of London, 29/39 Brunswick Square, London WC1N 1AX (0171 753 5800)
- Manchester: Department of Pharmacy, University of Manchester, Oxford Road, Manchester M13 9PL (0161 275 2411)
- Nottingham: School of Pharmacy, University of Nottingham, University Park, Nottingham NG7 2RD (0115 951 5052)
- Portsmouth: School of Pharmacy and Biomedical Science, University of Portsmouth, St Michael's Building, White Swan Road, Portsmouth PO1 2DT (01705 843 683)
- Strathclyde: School of Pharmacy, University of Strathclyde, Glasgow G1 1XW (0141 552 4400)
- Sunderland: Pharmacy Department, School of Health Sciences, Fleming Building, University of Sunderland, Sunderland SR1 3SD (0191 515 2582).

Infrastructure for dissemination of information and findings

Journals

Journals that have a record of publishing research on primary care pharmacy include:

- *British Journal of General Practice*
- *British Medical Journal*
- *International Journal of Pharmacy Practice*
- *Journal of Social and Administrative Pharmacy*
- *Pharmaceutical Journal*
- *Sociology of Health and Illness*
- *Social Science and Medicine.*

Conferences

The principal conferences and workshops for presenting primary care pharmacy research are:

- British Pharmaceutical Conference
- Health Services Research and Pharmacy Practice Conference
- International Pharmaceutical Federation (FIP) Congress
- Social Pharmacy Workshop.

SUMMARY

It can be concluded that, to date, primary care pharmacy research has largely failed to examine pharmacy services fully, has used suboptimal methodologies and has failed to explore how the provision of such services may be developed. However, for those wishing to research in this area there are numerous information sites available as a resource by any researcher considering an investigation in primary care pharmacy. The rapidly changing health service and the growing interest in primary care pharmacy as a legitimate area of study, suggest that primary care pharmacy research will prove fruitful area for future, detailed, rigorous research.

Personal experiences

INTRODUCTION

This section is based on our experiences of working together over the past ten years during which we have conducted several research projects, including studies of the relations between primary care pharmacists and general practitioners,[6,8] and the provision of injecting equipment to drug users from community pharmacies.[9,10] Our research experience has thrown up a number of methodological and pragmatic issues which may inform future research in primary care pharmacy.

Contacting and recruiting pharmacists

To recruit subjects to studies involving primary care pharmacists, researchers will need access to lists of community pharmacies or pharmacists. The Royal Pharmaceutical Society publishes annually, a full list of all registered pharmacists and community pharmacies in Great Britain, while each local health authority holds an up-to-date list of all pharmacies in their administrative area contracted with the NHS.

In our experience, pharmacists responsible for the management of the pharmacy are usually willing to participate in research if due care and attention is paid to their circumstances. However, when proposing to interview this group, researchers should be aware that in most pharmacies, the opportunity for interviewing pharmacists will be linked to the opening hours of the nearby GP practices. Clearly the period during and after surgery opening times will be particularly busy as patients present their prescriptions for dispensing. Similarly, a greater volume of prescriptions is presented at the pharmacy towards the end of the week. While it may not be possible to speak of an optimal time, when arranging to interview pharmacists, the end of the week and the opening hours of neighbouring GP surgeries should be avoided as far as possible. Also the last day of the month and the first two or three days are best avoided because of the administrative demands of processing each month's prescriptions for pricing by the Prescription Pricing Authority. These issues are particularly important for small pharmacies having only one pharmacist present on the premises at any one time.

Commercial nature of pharmacy and its impact on pharmacists' participation in research

Independent pharmacy contractors are essentially business people whose income derives from NHS remuneration for prescription services and profit from the sale of merchandise. Their participation in research projects, frequently by way of interviews and/or self-completed questionnaires is thus an intrusion, potentially impacting on their business. Pharmacists, like GPs, receive a considerable volume of unsolicited mail (of which self-completed questionnaires are one example) – hence the need to ensure a questionnaire that stands out and is enticing. Clearly the response rate is crucially important if the results are to be considered generalisable. There are several ways of ensuring an optimum response rate beyond the obvious prepaid reply envelope and a coherent user-friendly questionnaire. Offering respondents a copy of the final report is one option, and an innovative method we were associated with involved the researcher (a pharmacist) entering all completed and returned questionnaires in a prize-draw – the prize being one day's free locum cover provided by the researcher.

Adjacent pharmacies are as much competitors as colleagues. Pharmacists, when presented with a self-completed questionnaire, are thus unlikely to reveal commercially sensitive information such as prescription turnover, even when assured that such information will be treated in confidence and not used for any commercial purpose. One way round this, though far from ideal, is to offer a numerical banding from which pharmacists select their pharmacy's approximate prescription turnover. However, there is no reliable way of validating this information and it is perhaps best avoided. An alternative strategy might be to use a proxy measure, such as the number of full-time dispensing staff and/or number of pharmacists, size of dispensing area, etc., which indirectly indicates the capacity of the pharmacy for dealing effectively with large numbers of prescriptions.

MULTIPLICITY OF PRIMARY CARE PHARMACY OUTLETS

Given the heterogeneous nature of pharmacy outlets, unless the researcher wishes to access only one type of pharmacy, then stratified sampling is necessary to ensure representativeness. However, the participation of employee pharmacists in research projects invariably depends on clearance to do so from their line manager. In the case of the large multiples this requires the researcher to seek initial approval for the project in principle from the head office. This having been granted, approval from the pharmacists themselves must be sought. If approval is not secured from the large multiples, excluding them from the survey, it becomes impossible to generalise from the results.

AUTONOMY IN DECISION MAKING

Given the variety of primary care pharmacy settings, researchers should be aware that policy decisions within the pharmacy may emanate from a variety of sources and should therefore be interpreted with caution. For instance, when a pharmacist says that they do not supply injecting equipment to drug misusers, it is necessary for the researcher to explore whether this reflects company policy or the individual pharmacist's policy.

PATIENTS AS CUSTOMERS

Unlike other members of the primary care team, primary care pharmacists provide a commercial service to individuals as customers as well as patients. Despite reports of considerable customer loyalty – 62% of high users of primary care pharmacies tend to use only one pharmacy[11] – and the proliferation of patient medication records in pharmacies, it remains the case that primary care pharmaceutical services are provided to individuals as customers. A high-street pharmacy will serve a constantly changing and widespread population because of its location. Consequently, GPs and pharmacists do not share a defined patient population. Therefore researchers should be mindful of the fact that health-seeking behaviour will carry with it differential expectations when carried out in a GP's surgery, compared with a pharmacy, and this may be reflected in individuals' expectations and attitudes when seeking health services.

DIFFERENTIAL PERSPECTIVES OF GP–PHARMACIST RELATIONSHIPS

Pharmacists have traditionally been the handmaidens to GPs because they have less control over the prescribing/dispensing process, decisions as to who has medicines, how and when, being in the control of the prescriber. One implication of this differential relationship was evident in our experience of interviewing GPs and pharmacists. When asked to describe their relationship with one another, pharmacists were more limited in their expectations of the relationship. The result of this was that the word 'satisfactory', when used to describe their relationship, meant different things to GPs and to pharmacists. Therefore it should not be assumed that GPs and pharmacists, even when apparently collaborating together, share the same values, attitudes or even vocabulary to describe their relationship.

PHYSICAL AND GEOGRAPHICAL ISOLATION/SEPARATION

The physical separation of pharmacists from GPs (and indeed other members of the primary healthcare team) may act as a barrier to a mutual appreciation of their respective roles and functions and undermines the potential of any collaboration or team-building. Pharmacists are peripheral to the primary care team in the physical sense, which in turn mitigates the development of full cooperation and integration. Therefore it is important not to idealise the potential for cooperation, but to address the practicalities and the hurdles to the fostering of cooperation. For example, can a pharmacist wishing to speak with a prescriber access the GP directly without going through an intermediary such as the receptionist, and to what extent is this the case when the GP rings the pharmacy?

THE IMPORTANCE OF CROSS-DISCIPLINE COLLABORATION

We have discovered many advantages to working together as a medical sociologist and pharmacist on research projects. Intellectually, such collaboration is stimulating, because a single research question can be addressed from very different perspectives as each brings to that question different research skills and theoretical assumptions. This type of collaboration in primary care research also has a number of practical advantages, including the following.

New sources of information are revealed

A number of dedicated information sources, such as the libraries of the Royal Pharmaceutical Society and the Royal College of General Practitioners, restrict the range of their services for non-members. By collaborating with the appropriate healthcare professional researchers from the social sciences may gain access to these otherwise excluded resources by proxy.

Enhanced credibility

All primary care professionals routinely use abbreviations and acronyms, e.g. PMRs (Patient Medication Records), POMs (Prescription only Medicines). Clearly it is an advantage for collaborative researchers of primary care pharmacy to include a pharmacist who can key into the jargon. Similarly, our experience of cross-discipline collaboration has ensured that sociological jargon is avoided. This is especially important because it can raise suspicions regarding the purpose and relevance of the research from the perspective of primary care providers.

Raising the credibility of primary care pharmacy research

Much of the research that has been completed in primary care pharmacy has not been methodologically sophisticated and thus lacks credibility outside the immediate sphere of pharmacy itself. However, with the uptake and application of appropriate social science methods in primary care pharmacy research, more reflective and penetrating methodological analyses are being conducted, with a commensurate rise in the quality and status of this type of research.

Method and theory in research

Pharmacists' training focuses on their understanding of theories and methods within the framework of the natural sciences. Thus, they are not generally equipped to conduct the type of social research which commonly characterises a considerable bulk of primary care pharmacy research. Collaboration with social scientists can therefore enhance such research by:

- enabling primary care pharmacy research to explore, rather than treat as unproblematic, common assumptions shared among pharmacists, for example about individuals' health-seeking behaviour
- moving beyond a purely empirical level of data analysis by introducing a theoretical interpretation/dimension
- promoting a range of methodological techniques suitable for primary care research including quantitative and qualitative methods.

Personal factors

Collaboration across disciplines in an integrated sense, i.e. interdisciplinary rather than multidisciplinary, has, in our experience at least, led to developments that may not have been possible had we not purposefully sought to develop a research perspective on primary care pharmacy that drew equally on the social sciences and the agenda of pharmacy. Our efforts have not involved simply applying a social science perspective to research issues in pharmacy – this, in our minds, is the exclusive province of the social sciences. Nor have we sought to dilute the theory and methods of social sciences to make them more acceptable in an applied setting. Instead, we have attempted to develop a middle ground where social science perspectives are fully integrated within the agenda of primary care pharmacy research. It is neither purely empirical nor overly theoretical, but rather a blend of the two.

This has had several benefits:

- it has allowed us insights into primary care pharmacy which have derived from broad based theorising rather than descriptive empiricism
- it provides a more critical perspective on primary care pharmacy research than has hitherto been the case.

Summary

We have highlighted a number of issues that should be addressed when devising a research protocol for primary care pharmacy research to ensure the success and validity of that research. It is our experience that pharmacists are willing to participate in this research if the study is of demonstrable relevance and rigour, and investigators are reasonably cognisant of how pharmacists work in practice. We have found that cross-disciplinary collaboration is an effective and fulfilling means of ensuring this.

References

1. Nuffield Committee of Inquiry into Pharmacy (1986) *Pharmacy: a report to the Nuffield Foundation*. Nuffield Foundation, London.

2. Mays N (1994) *Health Services Research in Pharmacy: a critical personal review*. Pharmacy Practice Resource Centre, Manchester.

3. Woodward J (1992) GPs and community pharmacists – a study of attitudes. *Pharmaceutical Journal*. **249**: 99–101.

4. Bond CM, Sinclair HK, Taylor RJ *et al.* (1995) Pharmacists: a resource for general practice? *International Journal of Pharmacy Practice*. **3**: 85–90.

5. Spencer JA and Edwards C (1992) Pharmacy beyond the dispensary: general practitioners' views. *BMJ*. **304**: 1670–2.

6. Harding G and Taylor KMG (1990) Professional relationships between general practitioners and pharmacists in health centres. *British Journal of General Practice*. **40**: 464–6.

7. Royal Pharmaceutical Society of Great Britain (1997) *New Age for Pharmacy Practice Research: promoting evidence based practice in pharmacy*. The Report of the Pharmacy Practice R and D Task Force. Royal Pharmaceutical Society of Great Britain, London.

8. Harding G, Taylor KMG and Nettleton S (1994) Working for health: interprofessional relations in health centres. In: *Social Pharmacy: innovation and development* (eds G Harding, S Nettleton and K Taylor), Pharmaceutical Press, London, pp. 44–56.

9. Harding G and Taylor KMG (1991) Community pharmacists and HIV transmission reduction. *International Journal of Pharmacy Practice*. **1**: 102–6.

10. Harding G, Smith FJ and Taylor KMG (1992) Injecting drug misusers – pharmacists' attitudes. *Journal of Social and Administrative Pharmacy*. **9**: 35–41.

11. MEL Research (1991) *Consumer Expectations of Community Pharmaceutical Services. A research report to the Department of Health. Final report*. Aston University, Birmingham.

FURTHER READING

Mays N (1994) *Health Services Research in Pharmacy: a critical personal review.* Pharmacy Practice Resource Centre, Manchester.

Harding G Nettleton S and Taylor K (eds) (1994) *Social Pharmacy: innovation and development.* Pharmaceutical Press, London.

Soothill K, Webb C and Mackay L (eds) (1995) *Interprofessional Relations in Health Care.* Edward Arnold, Sevenoaks.

19

Social science research and researchers in primary care

Madeleine Gantley and Geoffrey Harding

THE THEORY

This section falls into two parts. The first details what might be considered primary care perspectives on what general practice and primary care researchers may believe social science can bring to primary care. The second presents our understanding of why social scientists value the research opportunities in primary care, which could also be interpreted, in our view, as why academic primary care needs social science. The divergence between the primary care and social science perspectives reflects the fact that social science and primary care operate with inherently different assumptions about issues relating to knowledge about health and healthcare. The distinction might be illustrated as a tension between a theoretically oriented discipline (social science) and an applied discipline, such as medicine, nursing or pharmacy, etc.

The primary care perspectives

Expanding the knowledge base of general practice and primary care

General practice has its origins in essentially reactive service provision, with occasional enthusiastic individuals active in local research. It has developed into both the proactive delivery of more holistic primary healthcare and the establishment of an academic discipline with its own distinctive research agenda. Academic departments of primary care undertake research on a range of topics, with a central theme of working towards the appropriate delivery of appropriate primary care, including the provision of information on the prevention of disease. As the scope of primary care has expanded over a range of fronts, for instance:

- policy change, such as the move towards a 'primary care-led NHS'
- developments in fields such as genetics
- the provision of an expanding range of services in primary care

so too the scope for research has broadened and the contribution of a variety of different perspectives has been sought.

Social scientists appear to be recruited to departments of general practice and primary care for a number of reasons:

- **Social science contribution to multidisciplinary and interdisciplinary research:** as the scope of primary care has expanded, so the range of professionals involved has expanded, e.g. community nurses and psychologists, and each has contributed towards an expansion in the potential primary care research agenda. With the increased emphasis on multidisciplinary and interdisciplinary research, the research base of the discipline has developed and has moved beyond the biomedical explanation of disease towards research acknowledging the importance of the patients' understanding of their health and the cause of disease; that is to say, research recognising that disease affects not only the body as a biological entity, but also the person as a social entity. It is only relatively recently that the social sciences, which are well qualified to contribute towards this type of understanding or explanation of health and illness, have been applied within general practice and primary care research. In doing so they have contributed towards the development of an academic base for general practice and primary care via multidisciplinary research which has aimed to broaden and deepen our understanding of healthcare delivery, health promotion, interpersonal communication and consultation skills. For instance, psychological theories have been drawn on extensively to shed light on human cognition and reasoning in relation to health behaviour, and sociological theories have been used to explain the existence and persistence of health inequalities. Thus the academic foundation is eclectic, drawing on insights from many other disciplines in pursuit of its broad – and constantly changing – range of objectives.

- **Social scientists as 'experts' on 'behaviour':** in the context of general practice and primary care, social scientists are frequently regarded as notional 'experts' in understanding people's social and psychologically determined behaviour. Certainly, social science has contributed significantly towards an understanding of the 'lay' perspectives on health, help-seeking behaviour and individuals' experience of illness. Psychologists in particular offer penetrating insights into the process of interpersonal communication, especially in the context of individuals' consultations with primary healthcare providers, and contrasting professional and lay explanations for illness causation and appropriate treatment.

- **Social scientists as methodologists:** as well as bringing a specialist body of knowledge which is directly applicable to primary care, social scientists also possess a range of social research skills and an awareness of, and often expertise in, a range of established methods from which to draw. These are frequently in demand within primary care settings, in contributing to the building of a multidisciplinary academic research base for general practice and primary care. Thus social scientists are regularly called on to assist in the design of survey research instruments or the collection and analysis of qualitative data, as well as to introduce analytical social science perspectives on the data.

- **Social science and primary care education:** social science has a clear role in helping to fulfil the General Medical Council recommendations about helping medical students understand the place of medicine, and the medical profession, in society, through their teaching input in departments of general practice and primary care, and in other areas of the medical curriculum. Moreover, at postgraduate level in particular, social scientists are able to bring to bear a critical view of knowledge and promote skills in critical appraisal of published research. Social science also has a high profile in the development of postgraduate taught degrees in primary care, as the traditional long-established definitions of health and healing, based on biological reductionism, are increasingly being complemented by socioenvironmental models, which explain health and illness as socially determined as well as biologically determined phenomena.

- **Social scientists as 'experts' in conceptual models of patients as consumers:** accompanying the NHS reforms of the early 1990s has been the development of a conceptual shift away from the idea of health (and ill health) as a consequence of fate, towards the concept of health as a commodity which, like all commodities, is increasingly also regarded as a resource of which one can have more or less. That is, individuals are increasingly exhorted to take responsibility for their own health and avoid unnecessary exposure to risk, through adopting specific lifestyle patterns. With this conceptual shift in understanding there has been a concomitant shift in the relationship between healthcare provider and recipient. Thus the traditional role of patient as passive recipient of care is increasingly being challenged by the emergence of the patient as active 'consumer' of health services. Social scientists in academic departments of general practice and primary care are thus called on to contribute towards measuring patient satisfaction with services, most often by the use of patient satisfaction surveys.

The social scientific perspective

For social scientists working in academic general practice and primary care there are many possibilities for research. They gain access to a source of rich research potential, among both the providers and users of primary healthcare services, which might otherwise be difficult to access. Moreover, these departments provide opportunities to explore the social construction of health knowledge and the dynamics of primary care delivery. Under this umbrella term there are a number of possible research topics from a social science perspective, including the following:

• The development of social theory-informed perspectives on the nature and dynamics of interpersonal relations among primary care personnel and patients, and the dynamics of the inter-relationship among these personnel. The issue of the patient–healthcare provider relationship is especially relevant as health and healthcare are increasingly perceived within consumer culture as a commodity of which one can have more or less, rather than as functions of biology and/or fate.
• Development of theoretical models of the nature of primary care teamworking, and the concept of leadership, team membership and the primary healthcare team itself. The relationship between various healthcare providers is especially important given the shift towards a primary care-led NHS.
• The organisation of primary care health services, including the introduction of managers, generates an interest in the concepts of managerialism and organisational culture within the healthcare arena. These concepts form part of broader sociological debate on the relationship between professional and managerial status, in areas such as education and social services.
• Other changes affecting the organisation and status of the medical profession have been termed the 'McDonaldization of medicine'. Ritzer and Walczak[1] describe this as 'antitrust decisions, corporatization, conglomeration, bureaucratisation, technological change, unionization, and the rise of McDoctors (no appointment, walk-in medical facilities modelled after fast-food restaurants)'.
• The ways in which sociocultural factors influence access to appropriate health services. There is potential for research in areas such as contrasting understandings of the nature of health and illness, differential expectations of health services among cultural groups, which in turn relate to variations in patterns of use; patients' help-seeking strategies, for instance patients' rationales in choosing to consult a pharmacist, GP, counsellor or alternative therapist.
• A theoretical perspective on explanation for inequalities in health and healthcare. The Black report on inequalities in health and the ten year follow-up 'The Health Divide' reported on the patterns of disease across social classes and inequalities in access to healthcare, and identified a number of possible explanations.[2] Factors such as ethnicity and socioeconomic status are clearly significantly associated with access to and uptake of health services, yet an

understanding of the nature of their interaction is not fully developed. This is a topic to which social scientific research has much to contribute.

- Social scientists are able to bring a broader sociohistorical perspective to the development of western biomedicine, and specifically the nature of primary care. This includes differential status of knowledge systems (or epistemologies), for instance positivist and social constructivist approaches, which underpin western medicine, and particularly evidence-based medicine.

- Again from a sociohistorical perspective, researchers may address the changing nature of general practice, in the context of the increasing secularisation of society in which the GP may function simultaneously as a combination of healer, confidant and confessor, taking on the role previously occupied by the clergy. At the same time as the broadening of the GP role, the practice of medicine has become increasingly routinised and regulated, with GPs taking on functions of child surveillance, population screening and so on. Social scientists may interpret this as part of the broader processes of 'bureaucratisation' and 'proletarianisation' of medicine.

- The body itself has been a topic of research for anthropologists and sociologists, the former concentrating on the body as symbol and the latter on the body as a socially constructed phenomenon.[3] Both disciplines have research interests in the body and 'body boundaries' and the appropriate but culturally diverse ways in which body boundaries may be crossed by healthcare professionals.

WHAT IT'S LIKE IN PRACTICE

There are a number of inherent tensions for those social scientists who take a career step away from social science departments towards departments of general practice and primary care. These tensions result partly from the contrast between the cultures of these academic departments, and partly from a lack of shared understanding about role definitions and expertise.

The world of departments of social sciences

Social science departments train their students in both the substance and methods of their specific disciplines, for instance sociology, anthropology or social psychology. Academic staff members are responsible for planning and implementing teaching, focusing on both the core areas of the discipline and their own specialist research fields. Thus a social anthropologist may teach a central topic of the discipline, such as kinship studies, and may also run one or more focused courses on specialist areas, such as gendered anthropology or the cultural construction of disease. A sociologist may lead general courses on the nature of the nation-state or theoretical analyses of the class system, but may also offer specialist courses on theoretical perspectives of power. Such specialist courses generally reflect their own ongoing area of research, which contributes to expanding the knowledge base of the discipline. At undergraduate level, methodological issues are implicit rather than explicit; the primary focus of research is the theoretical evolution of the discipline rather than methodological development. It is at postgraduate level that students begin to focus extensively on research methodology, but such teaching is placed within the context of a discussion of the status and validity of knowledge – that is to say students begin to study epistemological issues. Knowledge itself is a subject for study and discussion, and any research method is considered in terms of its potential and limitations for shaping any knowledge that is produced.[4]

Tensions in the process of shifting from a department of social sciences to a department of general practice

Sociological work on the processes through which groups of students take on a new professional identity, known as 'professional socialisation', focuses on the ways in which such students become members of a group which holds a specific, often powerful, view of their shared identity and activities. In one widely cited phrase describing medical training, the process has been likened to: 'Passing through a mirror (to create) the sense of seeing the world in reverse'.[5]

The shift from social sciences to academic general practice or primary care has many similarities. The new academic environment offers very different perspectives on the worlds of health, illness and healing. From a social science interest in, for instance, the ways in which people understand, experience and make sense of 'dis-ease' in its broadest definition, working alongside colleagues qualified in medicine brings a perspective in which people – regardless of their state of health – become 'patients', and research is centred around either specific diseases or the delivery of care. In parallel, the social scientist loses his or her disciplinary identity, and becomes a 'non-medic'. Indeed, the annual scientific meeting of the Association of University Departments of General Practice hosts a meeting specifically for 'non-medics', which attracts participants with diverse disciplinary backgrounds including sociology, anthropology, psychology, mathematics, education, and so on.

Social science literature characteristically treats doctors as an 'elite', a powerful group with access to culturally valued knowledge and to economic and other cultural resources. In contrast, the view from within general practice and primary care portrays the GP as overworked, relatively poorly paid in comparison with some hospital colleagues, and facing increasing and diverse demands. These demands come from vociferous and sometimes aggressive patients, from the constant pressure to take on new knowledge, and new priorities imposed by both government and the General Medical Council. The construct of the powerful

GP and the powerless patient which underpins some analyses of GP–patient interactions has a very different interpretation from within. This is not to accept the idea of the GP as powerless, but rather to point out the contrasts in the disciplinary cultures.

The social scientist: insider or outsider?

For the social scientist, the immediate problem lies in the extent to which one 'goes native' (a term used by anthropologists to describe participant observers who take on, uncritically, the identity and role of those they are intending to study). Sociologists have contrasted the roles of sociology in medicine and sociology of medicine;[6] anthropologists have discussed the advantages and disadvantages of clinical and critical medical anthropology.[7] In both disciplines, the distinction lies between working within the priorities and assumptions of western biomedicine and its practitioners, and attempting to challenge some of these priorities and assumptions. The social scientist may elect to work within the medical model or to stand outside and to critique the role of the medical practitioner in perpetuating inequalities in access to intellectual or economic capital. Working within a medical school may be seen by some social scientists – often those in 'pure' social science departments – as contributing to the power of medical model by expanding the medically led research base at the expense of research led by the needs and priorities of users of the health service, or research focusing on the values attributed to other forms of healing.

The political economy of research

For many social scientists, the reality of seeking employment in research leads them to applied health services research, often in departments of general practice and primary care. These departments are well placed to attract funding, albeit for short-term work with little potential for theoretical development. Social scientists are often employed on short contracts, as data collectors and/or analysts, frequently with little input into the design or conceptual development of research. Thus the hierarchy of general practice, with the GP at the head of a team, supported by nursing and reception staff, is replicated in research, with social scientists in supporting roles. For social scientists, taking a step back from their involvement to look at the process in which they are involved, this is an example of the distinction between interdisciplinary and multidisciplinary working, with the former being an equal mutually beneficial relationship and the latter a more hierarchical enterprise.[8]

'You only want me for my methods'

As social scientists move into research in general practice and primary care, a distinction emerges between the way in which they see themselves, and the way in which they are seen by their medically trained colleagues. While social science training equips graduates with the theoretical perspectives and analytical techniques which enable them to develop insights into, for instance, the ways in which people might interpret and understand the experience of illness, they tend to be employed for their methodological expertise. Thus in medical environments, generic 'social scientists' or 'behavioural scientists' are frequently employed because they offer a range of quantitative and qualitative research skills.

The idea of a generic social behavioural scientist with qualitative or quantitative skills represents a view by academic general practice and primary care of social science as offering essentially methodological rather than analytical expertise. In anthropology, or interpretive sociology, research is undertaken to explore people's understanding of a particular concept or the assumptions they share about a process such as help-seeking; the methods are implicit rather than explicit. They are designed to encourage informants to reflect on their own views and entail reflection on the nature of the knowledge they are likely to produce. Thus the social scientist moving into a medical setting has to deal with an expectation of methodological expertise but little or no understanding of the epistemological assumptions associated with either qualitative or quantitative methods. Some social scientists use the term 'methodolatry' to describe the emphasis on methods at the expense of analytical rigour.[9]

The process of adjustment: challenges and opportunities

As well as offering a series of challenges to the social scientist, academic general practice and primary care settings offer many opportunities, both professional and personal. The process of adjustment is one of recognising how various disciplinary perspectives differ, and how and where they may coincide. In some ways it can be likened to viewing the same image through the close-up (empiricist) lens of general practice and the wide-angle (theoretical) lens of one of the social sciences. The confusion lies in the process of focusing, of recognising that each perspective has its own intrinsic value. For the social scientist this may mean attempting to retain the two perspectives simultaneously: on the one hand, working within shorter-term research frameworks, focusing on data collection and analysis for applied health services research; on the other hand, retaining links with home disciplines through attending relevant conferences and maintaining reading within appropriate literature, to protect disciplinary expertise and potentially to contribute to the sociological as well as the primary care literature base.

Maintaining a balance

If on a practical level the social scientist can attempt to retain a balance by recognising the distinction between the narrower empiricist agenda of health services research and the broader agenda of the social scientists, on a theoretical level there is potential for social scientists to develop their own research agenda. This only becomes possible when a department can support a 'critical mass' of social scientists, to facilitate intellectual debate and the development of research ideas. A lone social scientist in a department faces a difficult task in attempting to introduce unfamiliar, and often challenging, methods and theoretical perspectives.

Much social science literature characterises biomedicine and its practitioners as epitomising a positivist, reductionist view of the human body and the experience of illness. Working within a general practice and primary care environment, however, opens up for the social scientist the possibility of exploring primary healthcare practitioners' own views of biomedicine, and of health and healing. It offers opportunities for research about professional carers' own experiences and beliefs, and help-seeking behaviour. The medicine that is practised in primary care settings challenges many of the assumptions that are associated with biomedicine.[10] Patients seeking primary care are necessarily viewed within their social context; their individual experiences and beliefs are recognised as important in their decision to consult; some GPs dare to question the currently culturally powerful notions of 'evidence-based medicine'.

The social scientist thus has the chance to work within the culture of primary care, but also to stand at its margins and to reflect on the processes of the social construction of knowledge that constitutes academic primary care. The challenge lies in working within the 'cultural borderlands'[11] of medicine and social sciences, while maintaining a sense of personal identity and professional credibility within each setting.

REFERENCES

1. Ritzer G and Walczak G (1988) Rationalization and the deprofessionalisation of physicians. *Social Forces*. **67**: 1–22.

2. Black D, Whitehead M *et al.* (1988) *Inequalities in Health: The Black Report and the Health Divide*. Penguin, London. Reprinted in 1990.

3. Turner BS (1992) *Regulating Bodies: essays in medical sociology*. Routledge, London.

4. Hughes J (1990) *The Philosophy of Social Research*. Longman, London.

5. Becker H *et al.* (1961) *Boys in White: student culture in a medical school*. Chicago University Press, Chicago.

6. Strauss R (1957) The nature and status of medical sociology. *American Sociological Review*. **22**: 200–4.

7. Baer HA (1990) The possibilities and dilemmas of building bridges between critical medical anthropology and clinical anthropology: a discussion. *Social Science and Medicine.* **30**: 1011–13.

8. Gilbert L, Selikow T-A and Walker L (eds) (1994) *Inter-professional Relations in Health Care.* Edward Arnold: Sevenoaks.

9. Janesick VJ (1994) The dance of qualitative research: design, metaphor, methodolatry and meaning. In: *Handbook of Qualitative Research* (eds NK Denzin and YS Lincoln), Sage, London.

10. Gordon DR (1988) Tenacious assumptions in Western medicine. In: *Biomedicine Examined* (eds M Lock and DR Gordon), Kluwer, London.

11. Rosaldo R (1993) *Culture and Truth.* Routledge, London.

Index